CATASTROPHIC INJURIES IN SPORTS: AVOIDANCE STRATEGIES

Second Edition

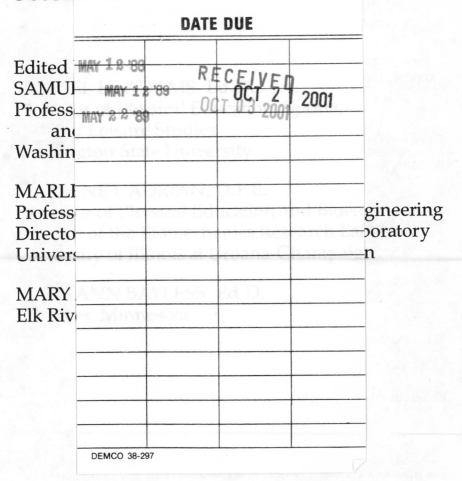

DATE DUE

MAY 18 '88		RECEIVED	
MAY 12 '89		OCT 29 2001	
MAY 22 '89			

Edited
SAMUE
Profess
and
Washin

MARLE
Profess ... gineering
Directo ...oratory
Univers ...n

MARY
Elk Riv

DEMCO 38-297

Benchmark Press, Inc.
Indianapolis, Indiana

Library of Congress Cataloging in Publication Data:

ADAMS, SAMUEL, 1928

CATASTROPHIC INJURIES IN SPORTS: AVOIDANCE STRATEGIES

Pages 251 through 254 are reprinted from: Fourth Annual National Gymnastic Catastrophic Injury Report, 1981-1982; Copyright 1983 by the United States Gymnastics Safety Association, Vienna, VA. Reprinted by permission.

Cover Design: Gary Schmitt

Library of Congress Catalog Card number: 86-72953

ISBN: 0-936157-15-1

Printed in the United States of America
10 9 8 7 6 5 4 3 2 1

The Publisher, Editors, and Contributors disclaim responsibility for any adverse effects or consequences from the misapplication or injudicious use of the information contained within this text.

Contents

PART IV ASSESSMENT, REPORTING, AND LITIGATION

Acknowledgements

The editors wish to express their appreciation to Trudy Haversat and Gary Breschini of Coyote Press, in Salinas, California, who published the first edition of this work.

Preface

Catastrophic injuries result in death, paraplegia, quadriplegia, and blindness. These are devastating not only to those who are injured, but also to their families and friends. Although the frequency of such injuries in sports is low, there is evidence that the numbers can be reduced. Research and public awareness programs have been two avenues for reducing the numbers of catastrophic injuries in sports.

Sports organizations, such as the United States Gymnastics Safety Association, have thoroughly studied the death and permanent neurological injury data in order to determine patterns of injury and preventative measures. Data banks and registries of sports injuries are available and provide additional information concerning catastrophic injuries.

Although most books about sports and the teaching of sports include some statements concerning safety and injury prevention, there is no single publication solely devoted to catastrophic injury prevention strategies for the teacher and coach of sports. This book represents such a publication.

Part I of this publication includes general information concerning liability, facilities and equipment, heat stress, and conditioning. Parts II and III consists of teaching and coaching strategies for avoidance of catastrophic injuries in 24 sports. Part IV consists of an action model for assessment of catastrophic injury potential, as well as general information concerning injury reporting, utilization of space, and a summary of litigation issues and strategy guidelines.

The coach, teacher, and administrator in sports should find this book useful as fundamental reading material to increase awareness of catastrophic injuries. Minimum reading should include Parts I and IV, along with the specific sport being taught or coached. Reading all the chapters will, of course, assist in developing a total perspective of the problem and in learning strategies to reduce the incidence of catastrophic injury.

Samuel H. Adams, Ed.D.
Marlene J. Adrian, D.P.E.
Mary Ann Bayless, Ed.D.

Part I

General Information

1

Liability and Negligence

SAMUEL H. ADAMS
Washington State University
Pullman, Washington

One of the American traditions which must rank alongside of apple pie and Chevrolet has changed in today's society. The tradition I'm speaking of is "not suing a coach." In past history, to even think of such a matter was sacrilegious, and a person who would think of doing such a deed was at least a heretic. However, tradition has changed immensely in the last 10 years, and lawsuits have changed the very nature of sport. There has been a significant redirection of lawsuits from product liability (suing a manufacturer of sports equipment) to suing coaches for their professional conduct.

Professional conduct of coaches is generally grouped into three areas: supervision, instruction, and responsibility for maintaining safe equipment and facilities. Professional conduct may be best defined as what the courts term "standard of care." Standard of care is the duty or responsibility to perform coaching duties effectively and properly. Although there are at present no set standards or competencies defining expected qualifications and performance of coaches, coaches are expected to have knowledge and competencies in order to act reasonably and prudently.

SUPERVISION

Supervision of student-athletes in sports is a critical area of responsibility. Negligence in this area can give rise to a lawsuit. There are two aspects of supervision—general and specific—that a coach must understand. General supervision indicates that the coach should be within the coaching area (on the field, in the gym) overseeing the activity, while specific supervision implies being at a specific location of activity (conducting a drill, conducting a scrimmage) with the student-athletes. Although it is not the intent of this book to delve into the supervisory responsibilities to which a coach should attend in avoiding liability suits, some identification of the two areas of supervision should be mentioned.

General supervision includes three definite responsibilities. These responsibilities are: 1) being able to oversee the entire program and immediately get to anyone who needs assistance; 2) being alert to conditions that may be dangerous to participants (defective equipment, poor or faulty facilities, discipline and control of participants); and 3) providing adequate and systematic first aid and emergency care.

Specific supervision involves knowledge of both the sport and the student-athletes and their capacity to do the sport or particular drill or activity. It also involves adhering to safety practices and procedures. A very important area of supervision is the appreciation of risk involved in the sport. The risks of the sport must be made known in very specific terms by the coach. A student-athlete does not assume any risks he/she is not aware of and does not appreciate.

MAINTENANCE OF EQUIPMENT AND FACILITIES

A discussion of maintenance of equipment and facilities is presented in Chapter 2 of this publication.

INSTRUCTION

Until recently, instruction by coaches was not questioned. Although some elements of instruction appeared to be highly risky and dangerous, they were accepted as part of teaching "mental" or "physical" toughness. For instance, in the past coaches denied players water breaks, even on extremely hot and humid days, to teach mental toughness. Football coaches employed dangerous drills such as a "suicide" drill where five to six players would tackle an unprotected lineman because he missed a block on an opponent who in turn had tackled the quarterback. These are examples of less than reasonable or prudent conduct obviously dangerous to the athletes. Coaches are likely to be sued for such behavior.

Another area of instruction in which the coach may be sued for negligence or unreasonable behavior is in the teaching of a skill or technique. A competent coach should know how to correctly and safely perform a skill or technique and how to teach each in a correct manner. These skills/techniques must be demonstrated and explicitly explained with respect to correct execution: how and what not to do, why an athlete needs to perform correctly, and the possible consequences of incorrect performance. Instruction must include the type of injuries that can occur, the nature of injuries that result, how the injury can occur, and how the injuries can be avoided (by using correct technique).

Coaches are considered experts in their sports and, therefore, are expected to use progression in both conditioning and development in skill/techniques. Before higher level movements or skills are attempted, lower movements and skills must have been taught and mastered. For example, a leaping forward roll is usually taught after the basic kneeling forward roll and then a standing roll are mastered. A fundamental understanding of arm and hand position, necessity of the tucked head, and an understanding of why these components are necessary to safely and successfully complete a forward roll must be prerequisites to the leaping forward roll.

If there are specific safety rules relevant to a skill/technique, these must also be taught and understood. This includes such instructions as the use of spotters in weight training and gymnastics and the difference between legal and illegal play. If an athlete were taught to perform an illegal skill, such as clipping in football, the person who taught him/her would be liable.

FORESEEABILITY

Foreseeability has become an element of negligence as an expected duty or standard of care for coaches. This was vividly pointed out in a case in the state of Washington where a coach and school district were sued for an injury that severely injured a football player. The allegations toward the coach and staff were as follows:

1. Failing to teach or instruct players not to lower their heads:
   A. to make contact with an opposing player using the head as a battering ram.
   B. to make contact with an opposing player such that it would remove any instinctive urge to do so.
   C. to utilize the helmet as the primary point of contact, and failure to affirmatively and positively teach players not to use such techniques.
2. Coaches did not read the points of emphasis section in the 1975 National Federation Football Rule Book to backfield players.
3. Coaches did not give out written materials relating to neck and spinal cord injuries or prevention of such injuries, nor did they show films, nor did they show photographs or diagrams, nor did they give demonstrations.
4. Failure to instruct as to how football players should position their heads at the time of contact with opponents.
5. Failure to warn as to the following:
   A. the dangers of head down contact.
   B. the mechanism of spinal cord injuries to players.
   C. initial contact with an opponent with the top of the helmet

while the neck is in flexion could result in injury to the spinal cord.

D. same as above except could result in quadriplegia.

The contentions of negligence directed to the school district included:

1. Failure to have coaches certified.
2. Failure to adopt rules that would prohibit a ball carrier from using the top of his helmet as an initial point of contact with another player.
3. Failure to adopt training rules such that players would avoid using their helmets as initial points of contact.
4. Failing to adopt a program for conditioning such players to avoid using their helmets as additional points of contact.
5. Failure to communicate to the coaches the medical, scientific, and statistical knowledge concerning the use of the head as a battering ram.
6. Failure to have a policy relating to instruction of matters concerned with safety for football coaches.
7. School district did not make mandatory injury prevention techniques by coaches to football players.
8. Failure of the school district to provide information to the players and parents of players concerning the physical risks to students participating in varsity football programs.
9. Failure to have a person in the central administration who had the responsibility for identifying risk to students participating as players in the varsity football program.

Most of the allegations toward the coach and staff and many of the ones against the school district either directly or indirectly involve foreseeability of possible injuries in the sport. Therefore, whenever an injury does occur, courts are asking:

1. Was the injury foreseeable? Should the coach have been able to foresee the incident and likelihood of the injury?
2. Could the injury have been prevented by warning the athlete? Were the risks involved in the sport communicated to the extent that the athlete understood and appreciated the risks?

It is important to note that knowledge of a risk is insufficient; there must be an understanding and an appreciation of that risk. An individual assumes only those risks of which he/she is knowledgeable and could appreciate. The knowledgeability and appreciation of risk assumes the fact that the inexperienced participant requires greater effort by coaches to communicate the risks involved. It also assumes that a prudent and careful coach would devote more coaching time in introducing new skills or activities to participants. However, if a participant is young but experienced, he/she is held to assume those risks of which he/she is knowledgeable and could appreciate.

The risks participants assume are those normal to the sport itself. Participants have the right to expect that equipment and facilities are in proper condition and that the instruction given is correct. When this is not true, these become negligent acts and participants do not assume any risks due to negligence. A person never gives license to anyone to be negligent at his/her expense. The signing of waivers or permission slips by parents simply means that the participant assumes the normal risks of a sport. It does not give permission for a coach to be negligent.

The major effect of what courts are ruling concerning foreseeability will be that coaches should know and identify major catastrophic injuries that could occur in each sport. They will need to know these injuries and have them in written form, and prepare plans for teaching safety factors, including diagrams and photos, demonstrations, and handouts.

This book deals with foreseeing catastrophic injuries and instruction in avoiding them. The authors of the different sections do not claim to identify all catastrophic injuries that may occur in a sport, but they do attempt to identify some of the most prevalent ones. They offer some suggestions to help avoid catastrophic injuries by proper instruction.

2

Safe Sports Equipment and Facilities

KENNETH A. PENMAN
Senior Associate; Associates in Education and Sport Research
Auburn, Washington

As with coaching and teaching sports skills, litigation involving a sports facility and/or an article of sports equipment is usually initiated by the occurrence of an injury. There are four basic reasons that injuries occur when participants use sports facilities: 1) the facility may be inadequately maintained (e.g., improper chemical balance of pool water, or moisture on a playing surface); 2) the facility may have been improperly designed and therefore is unsafe for certain activities (e.g., gym walls too close to court boundaries, or courts located too close to one another); 3) the facility may have a product associated with it which is defective (e.g., a synthetic surface that was not properly installed or is in a state of extreme wear); and 4) there is an inherent risk of injury while participating in any sports area.

The construction of a facility used to teach sports can be designed in such a way as to actually promote unsafe conditions. Playing surfaces with cracks, uneven joints, air pockets, and/or depressions may complicate a player's ability to avoid injury. Pools designed with inadequate depths, surface markings, irregular shapes, and slippery surfaces can cause injury.

Indoors, the most frequent cause of injury is insufficient clearance around courts. Baselines are often too close to walls, and walls are insufficiently padded. Objects such as benches and drinking fountains may be located too near the playing area for safety. Too frequently, gymnasiums have been built with glass windows and/or doors that were too close to playing surfaces. Numerous serious accidents have occurred as a result of participants crashing through glass surfaces. Uncontrolled building temperature and humidity, and inadequate lighting can also contribute to injury.

There are four basic reasons that injuries occur when participants use sports equipment: 1) the person is not supposed to be using the equipment, 2) an instructor has not shown the person how to safely use the equipment, 3) the equipment was defective in its production, and 4) the equipment is worn out and the instructor or coach has failed to recognize the inadequate condition.

In sports situations, equipment can be a lethal "weapon" and has to be carefully inspected to make sure there are no imperfections before it is used. For example, a bat can cause severe brain damage and/or kill an individual if it is defective and breaks at a crucial time. A hockey, baseball, or football helmet that is defective may lead to serious head injury. A foil can break and penetrate a fencing mask, and so on.

GENERAL PREVENTION MEASURES

1. Use recommended standards when designing a sports facility. If deviation from recommended standards has been made, have documentation as to why the modification is "safer."
2. Use common sense when designing facilities. Don't place glass surfaces, guy wires, poles, sprinkler heads, or sharp or blind corners near areas where vigorous activity is conducted.
3. Anticipate potential safety problems at the design stage. Have a safety officer and sports facility design consultant review plans, looking for potential safety problems.
4. Purchase quality building products and accessories, such as bleachers and standards, from reputable dealers who are noted for guaranteeing their products and providing good service to their customers.
5. Purchase quality sports equipment from reputable dealers who will "stand behind" their products.
6. For all existing facilities, designate a safety officer. Develop a clear written policy for establishing responsibility for inspection, maintenance, and reporting of safety violations related to sports facilities.
7. Designate someone to be responsible for regular inspection of sports equipment, and immediately remove defective and/or worn equipment from use.
8. Conduct periodic safety inspections, and correct unsafe situations by either taking those facilities out of use and/or placing warning signs in appropriate areas.
9. Keep accurate records of safety audits, correction of potentially unsafe facilities, and accidental injuries sustained within each sports facility.
10. Keep records of injuries related to equipment.

SOME SPECIFIC PREVENTION MEASURES

1. Make sure that protective equipment is kept in good condition and fits each student properly.
2. Refrain from "handing down" worn or defective equipment to junior varsity, freshman, and junior high teams.
3. Make sure that students are wearing protective gear as specified by the rules for the sport (i.e., mouthpiece in football).
4. Constantly examine equipment used in sports contests, such as bats, sticks, and racquets, to be sure they are free from defects that could cause injury.
5. Constantly watch for broken glass, moisture, and other materials on sports surfaces that could cause injury, and either remove the hazard or place the facility off limits until the condition is remedied.
6. Provide adequate storage facilities for locating sports equipment when it is not being used.

There is often a "fine line" drawn as to whether an injury occurs because of a lack of proper instruction or supervision, or whether it was due to poor equipment or an inadequate facility. To avoid potential injury to athletes, it is essential to do everything possible to prevent injury—regardless of the cause! By following the prevention measures listed previously, injuries due to equipment or a facility can be reduced to a minimum.

3

Heat Illnesses

DOUG SEBOLD
Washington State University
Pullman, Washington

The human body reacts to heat stress in much the same way as it reacts to physiological and mechanical stress placed upon it during the state of exercise. The principles of homeostasis, adaptation, specificity of adaptation, and chronic adaptation are analogous in both situations, and a cursory review of the principles will clarify the similarities.

The principle of homeostasis confirms that the body would like to remain in a state of equilibrium not only internally but with the external environment. Naturally, the body prefers an internal temperature of 98.6 degrees Fahrenheit, a constant pressure, absence from infections and all other trauma, and a psychological state of wellness. Interestingly enough, exercise is one of the major upsetters of homeostasis.

The principle of adaptation reminds us that, within given parameters, the body will adjust to varying conditions if adjustment is required. A rather simple example of this principle is our ability to ingest or delete foods from our diets, resulting in gains or decreases of weight.

The third principle, specific adaptation, revolves around the body's ability to adapt to minute stimuli which cause very specific changes to occur. Our diet lends itself quite well to this principle. By changing our eating habits from two or three meals a day to five or six meals a day, while maintaining normal living patterns, we can be assured that we will experience a gain in weight. The body cannot metabolize the extra food, and therefore elects to store it as fat. Finally, the fourth principle, chronic adaptation, becomes paramount because our body will chronically adapt to the situation or environment over time and is unchangeable unless specificity in the opposite direction is initiated.

Problems of heat illnesses follow the basic physiological principles, because heat stress is a tremendous stimulus to the external and internal environments of the body. Heat illnesses have been categorized into heat cramps, heat asthenia, heat syncope, heat fatigue, heat exhaustion, and heatstroke. Closely associated with these illnesses are the attendant problems of dehydration and potassium depletion. A complete description of heat illnesses is presented since an understanding of the physiological responses of the body will aid the player and coach in recognizing minor problems before they grow to catastrophic proportions.

THE HEAT SYNDROME: SYMPTOMS AND FIRST AID

Although an exact continuum does not exist for all heat illnesses, the **heat cramp** appears to be the least severe and results in the muscles' inability to relax. Generally, the cramp may be caused by a lack of salt, potassium, or magnesium. It has been the author's experience that many early season "heat cramps" were actually muscle strains which may have been caused by the fatigue factor or muscular spasm due to sustained muscular contraction. Nevertheless, one must not rule out the possibility of low mineral levels when confronted with "heat cramp," and proper evaluation of the condition is extremely important.

Muscle cramps respond effectively by stretching the muscle or muscle group and by applying grip pressure over the full length of the muscle. Rest, continued stretching, and the intake of a teaspoon of salt in an eight-ounce glass of water will usually alleviate the condition in a very short period of time. An athlete who has suffered two episodes of cramping during a 30-minute period should be restricted from further activity for the day to prevent possible serious damage to the muscles.

Heat asthenia and **heat syncope** are conditions which elicit the similar symptoms of fatigue, weakness, headache, blurred vision, high pulse rate, heavy sweating, possible mental or physical inefficiency, a poor appetite, insomnia, and an elevated body temperature. These conditions are caused by environmental conditions of very high temperatures and extremely high humidity. First aid should be the immediate removal of the athlete from the extreme environment. Body fluids and minerals should be replaced by giving water initially followed by a salt solution of water. The athlete should be directed to rest and to continue fluid replacement of fruit juices and water.

Heat exhaustion may be divided into three conditions. Heat exhaustion caused by water depletion results from the athlete's body's inability to replenish and maintain the necessary fluid level. Heat exhaustion caused by too much salt in the system will cause the body to lose water and potassium. Heat exhaustion may also be caused by too little salt in the system.

The symptoms of heat exhaustion from water depletion are generally excessive thirst, xerostomia (dry mouth), fatigue, weakness, weight loss, elevated temperature, possible mental confusion, and, in the later stages, a lack of coordination, increased heart rate, and a reduction of sweating. These symptoms will usually follow a long period of profuse sweating when proper fluid intake recommendations are not followed or quite frequently will appear when weight loss is required over a brief period of time. Wrestlers often use profuse sweating as a means to "make weight." Obviously, this practice should be forbidden by coaches and sports medicine personnel.

Although the symptoms of water depletion, heat exhaustion, and salt depletion are similar, there are a few symptoms unique to salt depletion problems. The particular difference between the two conditions is a time factor which causes salt depletion to occur over a period of three to five days. In this situation, salt is slowly depleted due to prolonged sweating without adequate replacement. The symptoms will usually center around fatigue, weakness, muscle cramps, dizziness, headaches, nausea, possibly an elevated temperature, vomiting, diarrhea, and infrequently, blurred vision. These symptoms are directly caused by prolonged sweating, inadequate or no replacement of salt to the diet, and poor accommodation of the body to the environment. Additionally, a salt depletion heat illness condition usually results in the depletion of potassium, magnesium, calcium, and other electrolytes.

First aid for athletes with symptoms of water depletion is obvious. The athlete must be moved to a cooler environment, the clothes and/or equipment must be removed, and large amounts of water administered. Later, fruit juice is the fluid of choice because of its rich mineral content. The athlete should be restricted from any participation for at least 24 hours, and then very slowly reintroduced to the normal schedule.

Heatstroke is the most severe heat illness condition and is considered a medical emergency. When 50 percent of the body's fluids are depleted, the thermoregulatory system reacts by shutting down the sweating mechanism. This causes the body's temperature to increase very rapidly to over 105 degrees Fahrenheit. Rectal temperatures approaching 110 degrees Fahrenheit have been recorded in heatstroke victims.

Symptoms of heatstroke may include previously mentioned heat illness symptoms, but the condition of heatstroke may also have a sudden onset. Frequently, the victim exhibits hot, *dry* skin, even in the arm pit and groin area; vomiting; high pulse rate; higher than normal blood pressure; headache; weakness; vertigo; and unconsciousness. The key symptoms appear to be hot dry skin and unconsciousness or near unconsciousness.

Immediate treatment for heatstroke begins with recognition and signaling for emergency aid. If an ambulance or emergency rescue squad is unavailable, a move to the local hospital must be initiated. The athlete must be removed to a cooler environment and all clothes except undergarments discarded. Cooling of the body may be accomplished by several methods. Cold showers, iced water applied with towels, submersion in a long whirlpool, application of alcohol, and rubbing of chipped ice over the extremities are methods that have been used effectively.

If the opportunity to pack chipped ice behind the neck and arm pits and layering the ice around and over the body is available, cooling of the body will be much faster. Remember, the primary need is to reduce the high temperature and get the athlete to medical attention. Athletes having suffered a heatstroke will usually require seven to 14 days of recuperation before they return to their sport.

Figure 3-1 is the author's conceptualization of the heat illness cycle. W "H" A T E R is an acronym for Water, Humidity, Acclimatization, Temperature, Electrolytes, and Rest. These all play a major role in the prevention of heat illness and will be discussed in conjunction with other known methods of heat illness prevention.

PREVENTION OF HEAT ILLNESSES

Deaths of football players from 1968 to 1972 and from 1973 to 1978 gave us tremendous insight into heat illness problems. The American College Football Coaching Association released statistics which indicated 25 football deaths in the earlier time period and only four in the latter. What happened? The answer became apparent after cursory research regarding the use of WATER by coaches and trainers, on the recommendations of physicians. Finally, in most instances water was freely accessible to the players or regular water breaks were scheduled by the coaches. Water, freely administered, reduced the death count by 21 young athletes over a five-year period. This statistic is certainly high enough in status and importance to eliminate the age old tradition of withholding fluids for the purpose of achieving the conditioned state faster. It did not! It will not! It will only continue to kill young athletes. The practice must cease now!

Prevention of heat illness from dehydration may be enhanced by the knowledge of water loss sustained by the individual athlete. This may be simply accomplished by posting a weight chart in the locker room and insisting that weigh-in and weigh-out procedures be conducted by all athletes. Figure 3-2 depicts a common weight chart, but this should be varied to meet the needs of the coaches and athletes. A variation of the chart might be the inclusion of body fat measurement and/or the recording of specific strength or flexibility measures.

With the knowledge that a 3 percent loss of total body weight may seriously impair performance and place the body in jeopardy of heat

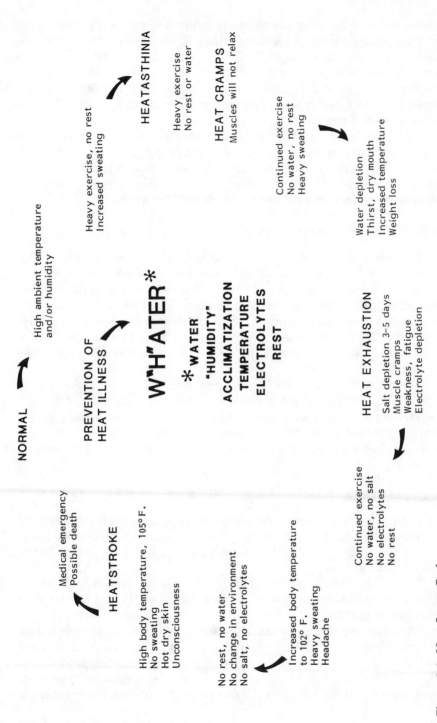

Figure 3-1. Heat Stress Cycle.

illness, the weight chart becomes an important gauge for identifying those individuals susceptible to any heat illness. Interestingly enough, there are the reports of football players losing 20 pounds or more in a two and a half hour practice session. Converted to fluid loss, this represents approximately 2.5 gallons. This reinforces the importance of required fluid replacement and free access to fluids during athletic competitions and practice.

Although heat illnesses have been more prevalent in football, they may occur in almost all sports. For example, fencing is a sport in which the body is covered in a manner comparable to that of football. Joggers may run in sweat suits on hot sunny days to reduce weight. Thus, the information in this chapter can be applied to all sports.

HUMIDITY, TEMPERATURE, AND WIND VELOCITY

Humidity, temperature, and wind velocity are factors which ultimately set the stage for heat illness problems. Difficulties arise in measuring true wind velocity, but all three factors may easily be determined by a phone call to the local weather station. Additionally, humidity and temperature may be measured by an instrument called a sling psychrometer. This device may be purchased at a medical supply house. Operating the psychrometer is quite simple, and the reading combines the wet and dry temperature.

Murphy and Ash (1965) have suggested the guide presented as Figure 3-3 for athletes requiring heavy equipment or clothing. Although the Wet Bulb Temperature is the most accurate measurement of the temperature and humidity environment, the knowledge of both separately has been calculated and procedures determined as suggested in Figure 3-4.

ACCLIMATIZATION

Acclimatization to heat and humidity is a natural phenomenon of the human body because of its exceptional adaptation processes. However, the body cannot adapt in an hour or day, but it will adapt to the environment in time.

Time is the commodity most often relegated to an inferior position. In the case of acclimatization for athletes, however, it must be placed in the superior position.

Various authors indicate that a minimum of three and a maximum of 10 days is required for the human body to adjust to extreme thermal conditions. Based upon the knowledge of acclimatization procedures, many professional, university, and high school conferences have mandated a period of time for football coaches to assure environmental ad-

Figure 3-2. Weight Loss Chart

Date

Sport

Time of Practice

Relative Humidity
Wet Bulb Temperature

ATHLETE:	% body fat	Wt. in	Wt. out	Loss	Wt. in	Wt. out	Loss

Figure 3-3. Wet Bulb Temperature Guide

Wet Bulb Temperature	Precautions
less than 60°F	No precaution necessary.
61° - 66°F 67° - 72°F	Alert observation of all squad members, particularly those who lose considerable weight. Insist water be given on field.
73° - 77°F	Alter practice schedule to provide rest periods every 30 minutes, in addition to the above precautions.
78°F or higher	Practice postponed or conducted in shorts.

Figure 3-4. Temperature/Humidity Guide

Temp. F	Humidity	Procedure
80° - 90°	Under 70%	Watch those athletes who tend toward obesity.
80° - 90°	Over 70%	Athletes should take a 10-minute rest every hour, and shirts should be changed when wet. All athletes should be under constant and careful supervision.
90° - 100° Over 100°	Over 70%	Under these conditions it would be well to suspend practice. A shortened program conducted in shorts and shirts could be established.

justment for the athletes. This may be an additional major factor in the recent reduction of heat illness deaths of football players.

A program of workouts beginning in the cooler times of the day and gradually progressing to the heat of the day is essential to prevent heat illness. The program may begin with workouts conducted in shorts and shirts in the morning and evening for a day or two. Additional clothing and equipment should be introduced gradually, and the workouts shifted to the heat of the day. Care must be taken to monitor environmental conditions since the Wet Bulb Temperature and Temperature/ Humidity Guidelines remain in effect. However, it is essential that workouts be conducted eventually at or near the time period in which games are played.

This may appear to be a difficult tight rope to walk, and it is! Therefore, to reduce the possibilities of injury, the athletes should be given an off-season conditioning program which includes workouts leading toward acclimatization prior to formal sessions.

Since clothing plays an important role in the dissipation of heat from the body, materials that allow evaporative cooling of the body should be worn. For example, it is imperative that meshed shirts and light-weight pants be worn by football players if at all possible. This minor requirement may pay heavy dividends in reducing heat illness. An excellent clue to the environment and the athlete's response to it is a completely soaked shirt of an athlete. This indicates profuse sweating and can only be seen after the shoulder pads are removed. These pads should be removed during the first "break" and a check of the shirts should determine the length of the break, the time of the next break, or an early conclusion or alteration of the practice schedule.

Finally, early session conditioning wind sprints need not be conducted in full gear. The athlete may be near water depletion, and the heavy exercise may be enough to initiate illness. Wind sprints in shorts will achieve the desired results.

ELECTROLYTES

The major electrolytes of the human body that are important in heat illnesses are sodium, chloride, potassium, magnesium, and calcium. These five electrolytes are especially important for the normal function of skeletal muscle in an atmosphere of adequate water.

Sodium chloride or table salt is lost during heavy sweating, but much more water is lost. In most instances, the athlete acquires more than enough salt in a normal diet and needs only to use a little extra at meal time during early season workouts. Athletes with weight losses of six pounds or more per practice session should consume one seven-grain salt tablet with one pint of water.

Potassium loss during heavy exercise may be replaced by the inclusion of bananas, leafy vegetables, molasses, and ketchup in the regular diet. Magnesium plus potassium are found in fruit juices, which should be the fluid of choice for all athletes. Calcium may be replenished to the system by ingesting milk and milk products. Numerous electrolyte drinks are available and most contain the necessary ingredients to replenish lost minerals.

Deaths from heat illness are definitely preventable by individuals in a supervisory role, because the information existing about the problem has been available for some time. Now is the time for the supervisors to acquire and implement the knowledge to assure future athletes lifelong enjoyment of sports.

PREVENTION OF HEAT ILLNESS, AN OUTLINE

(After Klafs and Arnheim 1981)

Environmental conduct of sports: particularly football.

I. **General Warning**
   A. Most adverse reactions to environmental heat and humidity occur during the first few days of training.
   B. It is necessary to become thoroughly acclimatized to heat to successfully compete in hot and/or humid environments.
   C. Occurrence of a heat injury indicates poor supervision of the sports program.

II. **Athletes Who Are Most Susceptible to Heat Injury**
   A. Individuals unaccustomed to working in the heat.
   B. Overweight individuals, particularly large linemen.
   C. Eager athletes who constantly compete at capacity.
   D. Ill athletes, having an infection, fever, or gastrointestinal disturbance.
   E. Athletes who receive immunization and subsequently develop temperature elevations.

III. **Prevention of Heat Injury**
   A. Take complete medical history and provide physical examination. Include:
      1. History of previous heat illnesses or fainting in the heat.
      2. Inquiry about sweating and peripheral vascular defects.
   B. Evaluate general physical condition.
      1. Type and duration of training activities for previous month.
         a. Extent of work in heat.
         b. General training activities.

C. Measure temperature and humidity on the practice or playing fields.
1. Make measurements before and during training or competitive sessions.
2. Adjust activity level to environmental conditions.
   a. Decrease activity if hot or humid.
   b. Eliminate unnecessary clothing when hot or humid.
D. Acclimatize athletes to heat gradually.
1. Acclimatization to heat requires work in the heat.
   a. Recommended type and variety of warm weather workouts for preseason training.
   b. Provide graduated training program for first seven to 10 days—and other abnormally hot or humid days.
2. Provide adequate rest intervals and salt and water replacement during the acclimatization period.
E. Body weight loss (water and salt loss) during activity in the heat.
1. Body water and salt losses should be replaced as they occur.
   a. Supply cold saline—thoroughly mix 1 teaspoon salt in 6 quarts of tap water—give three to four ounces every 15 minutes or eight ounces every half-hour.
   b. Allow additional water as desired by players.
   c. Provide salt on training tables and encourage salting of food.
   d. Weigh each day before and after training or competition.
      (1) Treat athlete who loses excessive weight each day.
      (2) Treat well-conditioned athlete who continues to lose weight for several days.
F. Clothing and uniforms.
1. Provide light-weight clothing that is loose fitting at the neck, waist, and sleeves. Use shorts and shirts at beginning of training.
2. Avoid excessive padding and taping.
3. Avoid use of long stockings, long sleeves, double jerseys, and other excess clothing.
4. Avoid use of rubberized clothing or sweatsuits.
5. Provide clean clothing daily–all items.
G. Provide rest periods to dissipate accumulated body heat.
1. Rest in cool, shaded area with some air movement.
2. Avoid hot brick walls or hot benches.
3. Loosen or remove jerseys or other garments.
4. Take saline and/or water during the rest period.

IV. Trouble Signs: Stop Activity!

Headache
Nausea
Mental slowness
Incoherence
Visual disturbance
Fatigue
Weakness
Unsteadiness
Collapse
Unconsciousness
Vomiting
Diarrhea
Cramps
Seizures
Rigidity
Weak, rapid pulse
Pallor
Flush
Faintness
Chill
Cyanotic appearance

4

Strength Training

BILL CHRISTIE
Washington State University
Pullman, Washington

Weight training has become an essential part of the preparation of athletes for optimal performance. The purpose of weight training for athletics is to develop strength, speed, and explosive power. This is accomplished through Power and Olympic lifting programs which may require the use of heavy weights and multi-jointed exercises.

Catastrophic injuries resulting from weight training should in fact be nonexistent. Weight training, when properly conducted, is one of the safest activities. Catastrophic injuries become a risk only in situations where carelessness and ignorance impair good judgment and common sense.

POSSIBLE CATASTROPHIC INJURIES

Types of possible catastrophic injuries that might occur during improper weight training are:

1. Suffocation may be caused by lifting without supervision or spotters. Attempting to lift heavy weights and losing control may result in a bar falling over the chest or throat. This may occur during the bench press.

2. Improper breathing is the *indirect* cause of concussion, brain damage, or death. It is the act of falling that produces the catastrophic injury. The fall is a result of fainting due to improper breathing. For example, if the breath is held or hyperventilation occurs to cause partial or complete loss of consciousness, the athlete may lose control of the weight bar and experience a catastrophic injury.

3. Loss of sight, brain damage, death, and other injuries may be caused by failing to use and secure collars on the bar. This

allows weights to slide off one end of an unbalanced bar, causing the other end to flip quickly in the other direction, possibly striking another person. This may occur with the bar on a rack or during any lift if the performer loses balance or control.

4. Damage to chest, including heart and lungs, and possible death may be caused by bouncing the weight off the chest to gain extra momentum in the bench press.

5. Possible damage to the spinal column may be caused by lifting heavy weights with improper technique and without spotters. This may occur during any heavy lift.

PREVENTION OF CATASTROPHIC INJURIES

The responsibility for injury prevention in a strength program lies with the instructor or coach. Beyond this, the administration should be held responsible for hiring or appointing instructors who possess thorough knowledge and understanding of the skills, techniques, progressions, programs, equipment, and safety requirements, as well as the organization and administration of a program.

Instructional Responsibility

A safe and successful program can be maintained through proper instruction and supervision. Instruction should begin with an orientation to the facility and equipment. This includes safety procedures for use and care of equipment, performance of exercises, behavior in the weight room, and possible dangers of improper use and performance.

The instructor should be educated in the scientific principles of strength training. Such books as Elam (1981), O'Shea (1969), Shepard (1977), Hooks (1974), and Wilmore (1982) are recommended reading.

Warning of Dangers
Instruction on safety and weight room conduct should include:

1. *Discipline and order in the weight room:* Do not allow wandering around the room. This disrupts others and leads to carelessness. Stay with each station and concentrate on it. All persons are as important to the safety and success of their partners as their partners are to them.

2. *Work in groups of 3-4:* There should be working groups of three to four members at each station. This helps keep the group organized and insures safety by having stoppers for each lifter. Lifting in isolation can lead to injury when using free weights and working with heavy loads, and therefore is not allowed.

3. *Proper use and care of equipment:* Equipment should always be put in its proper place when not in use. Loose weight equipment laying around the room can be hazardous and can lead to injury.

In a cluttered room, persons may trip and fall, possibly hitting their heads or other body parts. It is also important to report any faulty or damaged equipment to the instructor so it can be attended to quickly.

4. **Number of participants:** This will be determined by the size of the facility and the amount of equipment. Generally, there should be no more than three to four persons to a station, and there should be no one else in the room other than the instructors or supervisors.

5. **Use of collars:** Collars should be used at all times to secure the weights on the bars. Neglect can lead to serious injury, as a bar could have its weights slide off and flip over, hitting another person.

6. **Breathing:** Inhale to begin a lift and exhale before completing the lift. Holding the breath throughout a lift can cause the lifter to faint and fall and/or drop the weights on himself/herself.

7. **Spotting:** Use spotters for all free weight lifts. Spotters are lifting partners who help the lifter through any difficulty. Lifting without spotters is dangerous, and injury can result from losing control and having the weights fall or the lifter collapsing under the weight.

8. **Bouncing and jerking:** The athlete should not bounce or jerk the bar when performing a lift. The weight should be lifted with a tight and controlled movement. Bouncing off the chest (as in the bench press) can cause chest, lung, and heart damage. Jerking the weight to start a clean or deadlift can cause back or shoulders injury.

9. **Progression:** Master the techniques of the exercise using light weights before progressing to heavier weights. This allows for conditioning of the muscles and joints in preparation for more intense work. Lifting heavy weights with improper technique and lack of conditioning can cause injury to muscles, joints, and the spinal column.

PROPER INSTRUCTION AND CORRECT TECHNIQUE

Development of correct lifting techniques for each exercise is an important factor for injury prevention. The instructor must possess the knowledge and ability to teach the athletes these techniques. This can be accomplished through explanation, demonstration, and the use of instructional films.

Teaching technique is an ongoing process and requires constant supervision and coaching. It is the job of the instructor throughout the program to teach and help improve each athlete's technique. This in itself is a major safety feature.

The four most common exercises used in strength programs are the power clean, squat, bench press, and the deadlift. The correct techniques for performing these exercises are presented below.

Power Clean

Starting Position
1. Feet should be hip width apart with toes turned slightly out. Bar should be positioned over shoestrings.
2. Weight should be distributed over insteps of each foot with feet flat on floor.
3. Body should be in a semi-squat position with back and shoulders flat. Chest should be over the bar.
4. Hands should be shoulder width apart and using an overhand grip.

Initial Pull
1. The arms should be kept straight with elbows locked and shoulders tensed. The back and shoulders should remain flat and the abdomen tensed.
2. The weight should be "driven upward" with the legs. Hips should also rise vertically from the leg drive. Pull strongly and steadily—*not quickly*. (Do not jerk the bar off the floor.) Keep the head up and the back straight.
3. The initial pull should bring the bar to a position just above the knees.

Scoop and Power Pull
1. When the bar passes the knees, bring it back toward the thighs and simultaneously dip the hips.
2. To accelerate the bar, drive the hips (quickly) forward and upward, keeping the head up and the bar close to the body.
3. The body should be extended vertically (do not lean or pull back) all the way up on the toes.
4. When reaching full extension, shrug the shoulders, and pull the bar as high as possible, keeping elbows high and to the side.

Rack
1. When the bar is pulled to its highest point, snap the elbows forward and bend at the knees to bring the body under the bar.
2. The elbows are up and forward and the bar is positioned to rest on the front of the deltoids (rack position). When the bar is racked, stand up.

Lowering
1. Return weight from rack position to thighs, controlling the bar, keeping the back straight, and bending the knees. Return the weight to the floor in the starting position.

Squat

Starting Position
1. Feet should be slightly wider than the hips with the toes pointed slightly out.
2. The bar should be centered across the back resting on the notch formed by the back shoulder muscle. (Bar may also rests at base of neck.)
3. The head should be up, knees locked, back flat, and abdomen tensed.

Lowering the Weight
1. Take a deep breath and allow the knees to bend forward in line with the toes.
2. Squat slowly, controlling the weight to a position where the top of the thighs are near parallel with the floor. (When top of hip meets the thigh there should be a locking sensation.)
3. Do not bounce at the bottom position, as this can result in severe knee injuries.

The Upward Drive
1. Once in the bottom position, return to the upright position by "driving" strongly, utilizing a powerful hip and leg thrust (extension).
2. The back should be kept flat and tight to avoid any forward tilt. (Keeping the head up and forcing the neck back on the upward drive will help keep the back straight.)

Bench Press

Starting Position
1. Points of contact: feet on floor, hips on bench, head and shoulders on bench.
2. Back may be bridged between buttocks and upper back.
3. Grip bar with hands wider than shoulders and, using an overhand grip, squeeze bar tightly.

Lowering and Raising
1. Take a deep breath and lower bar to mid-chest, touching slightly, without bouncing.

2. Keeping tension on the floor with the feet, use a powerful arm, shoulder and chest action to push bar to an extended position.
3. Keep the buttocks on the bench—do not heave or arch.
4. Upon completing the upward drive, lock elbows to complete each repetition.

Deadlift

Starting Position
1. Feet should be about hip to shoulder width apart.
2. The overhand or alternating grip may be used. Hands should be the same width as for the power clean.
3. The bar should be positioned over the shoestrings, and the feet should be flat on the floor.
4. The shoulders should be out in front of the bar.
5. The back should be flat (extended), abdominal muscles tensed, and the arms straight (extended).

The Upward Drive
1. The movement should begin with a strong leg drive (extension).
2. During the first part of the movement, the back angle is maintained, and the hips rise vertically due to the extension of the legs.
3. The shoulders should be kept above and in line with the bar. This helps keep the hips close to the bar.
4. The hips are brought forward to get in line with the shoulders.
5. The back is extended until the shoulders are directly above the hips. It is not necessary to lean backwards at the completion of the movement.

PROGRESSION OF SKILLS

Progression in weight training must be thought of in terms of training phases (training at various intensities or workloads for given periods of time).

Programs generally consist of three or four core exercises which are complete movements or skills in themselves. Technique or skill for performing the lifts is best developed by using light weights (e.g., what the lifter can handle for eight to 12 repetitions) while concentrating on performing with correct technique, and gradually increasing weight as technique improves.

SPECIAL SAFETY CONSIDERATIONS

Facilities and Equipment

Designing a weight training facility requires several considerations for safety and efficiency. The size of the room should be adequate to allow operating space for all equipment. This includes enough space between stations to allow for free flow of traffic and for groups of three or four people to be working at each station. The ceiling should be 10 to 12 feet high to allow adequate room for overhead lifts and for adequate ventilation.

Each station should be equipped with storage racks to keep the weights in place when not in use. Racks should be firmly secured to the floor, or in the case of portable racks, should have a base large enough to prevent toppling when weights are loaded and unloaded on the rack. All weights and bars should have a specific place to be stored.

Platforms should be about eight feet by eight feet in size and should be placed in corners where possible. This reduces the number of open sides to two, which eliminates the possibility of someone coming up from behind a lifter and possibly being injured.

Maintenance of the facility is also an important safety consideration. The weight room should be kept clean, and all equipment should be in its proper place at all times. The equipment should be kept in good working order, and broken or faulty equipment should be replaced immediately.

There are also ergogenic aids and protective equipment available that should be present. There should be lifting belts for each power and Olympic station. These belts give support to the abdominal area and lower back. Each bar should be equipped with collars to secure the weights. Straps give support to the grip when working with heavy weights on the platform. Chalk is also used to aid the grip and help prevent blistering or soreness in the hands to avoid accidental dropping of the bar.

SPOTTING

The Squat

Three spotters are used. One is positioned behind the lifter and helps him or her through the "sticking point," if necessary, by gripping the bar and assisting upward. The other two spotters stand on the sides and don't touch the bar during the lift, unless called on to help. If the lifter starts to collapse at the bottom, they will catch the bar. The side spotters also help guide the lifter when returning the bar to the rack.

The Bench Press

There should be one spotter positioned behind and at the middle of the bar and a spotter on each end of the bar. The one behind the bar lifts the bar from the rack to the lifter and helps the lifter through the "sticking points" if he or she has trouble. The spotters at the sides help only when called on or if the bar starts to fall.

The Deadlift

There is only one spotter used for the deadlift. The spotter takes a position to the side and rear of the lifter. The rear hand is placed on the low back. The crook of the elbow of the other arm is placed over the front of the shoulder and the arm is under the chest. As the lifter begins the movement, the spotter gives a slight pull upward and backward, with the arm under the chest and a slight pressure on the back, to make sure the lifter stays in the proper position.

Part II

Team Sports

5

Baseball

RALPH DICK
University of New Mexico
Albuquerque, New Mexico

The description of the game of baseball is very similar to that of softball (Chapter 13), and the possible catastrophic injuries are similar (Table 5-1). The one thing that is different is the ball: it is smaller and harder than the softball. This means that the potential for catastrophic injury as a result of being struck by the ball in baseball is greater than it is in softball. Particular attention should be paid, then, to all circumstances where a player may be struck by a pitched, batted, or thrown ball. The possible catastrophic injuries in baseball are similar to those in softball. Refer to the list in Chapter 13.

PREVENTION OF CATASTROPHIC INJURIES

The warnings included in Chapter 13 are applicable to baseball. How they are emphasized may vary as the two games vary one from the other, but the communication of the warnings is no less important. More persons have died from being struck in the chest than from being struck in the head in these sports. In particular, protection of the chest and vital organs is important to batters.

CORRECT TECHNIQUE TO AVOID INJURY

The reader should refer to the chapter on softball for general guidelines concerning coaching strategies for developing the skills and knowledge necessary to avoid catastrophic injury-producing situations. Those aspects unique to baseball, or factors needing specific emphasis, are presented in this section.

Table 5-1. Possible Catastrophic Injuries in Baseball

Activity	Possible Injury	Cause	Prevention
Batting	Head injury, Brain injury, Loss of sight, Organ damage	Being struck by the ball	Batting helmet, Alertness, Knowledge of moving away from a pitch
Baserunning	Head injury, Neck or back injury	Hit by a thrown ball, Collision with defensive player	Knowledge and application of rules and strategy, Alertness
Sliding	Head, neck, back injury, organ injury	Collision with base or defensive player	Correct technique and appropriate use of skills
Fielding	Head or neck injury, Organ injury, Eye injury	Collision with another player or field obstacle, Being struck by the ball	Teamwork, "Calling" for the ball, Alertness, Appropriate positioning
Pitching	Head or eye injury	Being struck by a batted ball	Correct pitching technique and development of fielding skills

Batter Hit by Pitched Ball

Being struck in the head by a pitched ball can result in blindness, paralysis, coma, or even death. It is not a common occurrence, and there are several ways in which it can be reduced in frequency. The first is the hitter's personal knowledge of the pitcher, including mental makeup and control; knowledge of the opposition's general philosophy can help. In addition, the lighting system for night games can be adjusted so that the batter stands out well against a dark background. Batters should be taught to lower and turn their heads away from the ball and use the arms to cover their torsos. Emphasize specific practices in covering the torso. Ruptured spleens, stoppage of breathing from chest impacts, and kidney ruptures have been reported during baseball and softball play.

Protective padding for the torso is being manufactured. It should be evaluated by teachers and coaches with respect to use by players.

There are a number of drills which can be used to train hitters to deal with pitched balls. These are discussed briefly below:

Release point drill: The batter should concentrate on the ball as it is released from the pitcher's hand. The batter's goal will be to identify the release point while the pitcher is pitching (the batter will not swing at the ball). The goal is for the batter to see the ball as clearly as possible.

Calling the pitch drill: This is the same as the release point drill, but the batter's goal is to quickly identify the pitch. The batter calls out the pitch as it is identified.

Rolling with the pitch drill: In this drill the pitcher can throw from any distance, and uses a softer ball (Titus II or tennis ball). The batter reacts to the pitch. If it is a strike, it is to be hit; if it is at the body, the batter rolls the body with the pitch as it hits. This drill is designed to give the courage to hit the ball and to practice being hit in the body with the pitch.

Safety equipment needed: The hard hat is used while batting, but also protects the runner while on base.

Coaching points: Players must wear batting helmets whenever hitting, whether in a practice or a game situation. The coach must be sure that the helmets fit properly and should warn the players, with appropriate examples, of the potential for head injuries.

Pitcher Hit by Batted Ball

Being struck by a batted ball can result in broken bones, blindness, paralysis, coma, or even death. With the exception of the catcher, the pitcher is the closest defensive player to the batter, and many hard balls are hit toward the mound. Pitchers should know methods of self protection.

Techniques for pitcher protection: The pitcher should finish the pitch with the push off leg parallel to the stride leg. If the legs cross, the pitcher will have very little mobility and will be more vulnerable to a ball hit to the mound. Also, during the pitch the pitcher should use the glove arm in such a way that the glove is in front of the pitcher, and can field a returned ball.

Pitcher protection drills: Drills in which the ball is hit back to the pitcher should be organized. Also, pitchers can work on form, including position of the lead arm, with a partner or a mirror. The final position for fielding should be evaluated with respect to its ability for self protection. The lead arm must be used to turn the body into a fielding position (lead arm drill).

Coaching points: In general, the lead arm drill is badly under-coached. This is a fundamental for both safety and control, and it is as important as anything else in pitching fundamentals.

Injuries to Sliding Baserunners

While sliding, a player is susceptible to broken legs, broken fingers, arm, or wrist, concussion, and spike wounds. Some of these injuries can be reduced by teaching correct technique.

Bent leg slide: This is the most widely used slide in baseball; it is the safest, surest, and the fastest of the feet first slides. In sliding, the runner should try to keep the hands off the ground in order to keep from jamming wrists, although this sometimes provides an easier target to be tagged.

Bent leg drills: The slide should begin some eight to 12 feet from the base. Players should not slow down to begin the slide, or lean backwards going into the slide. The front leg should be held off the ground so that the spikes do not hit the ground. Players should not change their minds once they begin to slide. In drilling this technique, coaches should first cover the slide point by point, and in slow motion. Beginning players might begin by removing shoes and sliding on wet grass, using a loose bag or glove as the base. Players should progress at their own speeds until the fundamentals are attained. The actions can be gradually speeded up as confidence and skills develop.

Head first slide: The head first slide is faster and presents less of a target to the tag. It does, however, have a number of disadvantages; it is more dangerous because of the exposed upper body parts; the possibility of head or neck injury is greater; it can result in jammed fingers, wrists, and shoulders; and the runner cannot protect against falling infielders. This slide, in general, is harder on the body.

Head first drills: First, teach players never to slide into home plate with the head first, as the catcher is there with hard protective equipment. Head first drills are similar to bent leg drills. The slider takes the weight on the chest and stomach, and keeps the feet off the ground for less drag. The head is kept up to see where the ball goes, and the arms are extended toward the base. As in the bent leg drill, the runner should not slow down on the approach.

Infielder/Outfielder Collisions

Collisions between various infielders and outfielders can result in broken bones, concussion, coma, or even death. The players should be coached to be aggressive, but collisions occur when there is a lack of communication. There should be a standard communicating procedure established to cover all players. For example, the player who wants the ball calls "mine," while others involved yell "take it." Players calling for the ball should do so more than once. The outfielder has the right of way if both infielder and outfielder are going for the ball, but the outfielder should not attempt to call off any infielder who is standing underneath a pop-up near the infield. Finally, the fielder who is called off the ball should stay away from the fielder making the catch, so that the latter does not hear footsteps.

Coaching points: Establish the communication procedure on the first day of practice and use drills to make sure it is used. Inform the players of the importance of communication on pop-ups and the potential injuries which can occur.

Player Hit by the Bat or Batted Ball
While in the On-Deck Circle

Being struck by either the bat or a batted ball fouled into the on-deck circle can be cataclysmic or fatal. Alertness has been discussed. However, the person in the on-deck circle is in a particularly vulnerable position. Players should be instructed to always watch the pitched ball until the pitch is complete or the batter has hit the ball. Warm-up swings should be taken in between pitched balls so that full attention can be given to each pitch.

SPECIAL SAFETY CONSIDERATIONS

Field Layout

Not all coaches have a chance to have fields designed especially the way they want them, but most coaches have the opportunity to add safety features. The following are a few recommended safety features for baseball fields:

1. A warning track completely around the field. It should be 15 feet wide in the outfield and five feet wide the rest of the way around.
2. Build the dugouts as far away from the foul line as possible (preferably 60 feet).
3. Place the on-deck hitters' circle half way between dugouts and homeplate to reduce congestion around the dugout.
4. Place protective padding on areas of heavy use that present safety hazards.

Coaching points: Inform and show players how to use the warning track, and allow them to become familiar with the distance between the grass and the fence. Inform players in the dugout how to help infielders make catches near the dugout. Finally, warn the players of the dangers of walking through an area in which hitters are swinging bats without paying attention to their surroundings.

Catcher's Equipment

Catchers take pride in their equipment and how it fits. Shinguards and chest protectors should fit snugly, and adjustments should be made continually. Below is a list of catching gear and the problem areas to be aware of:

Mask: Securely snap the padding into the mask. Check the bars of the mask to make sure that none are broken. The mask must fit snugly and should not slide from side to side. Use a throat protector, and tie it in securely. Catchers should always wear hard hats or catcher's hard hats for protection from the free swinger.

Shinguards: Check the plastic portions for cracks, and make sure all elastic hooks are on each ring for a good fit. These elastic hooks should be pulled snug. Shinguards must fasten on the outside to keep from snagging when the catcher is running.

Chest protector: The chest protector must be snug against the throat for proper protection.

Cup: Males should never catch without a cup.

Coaching points: Outline the importance of properly fitting equipment and be sure that catchers check it periodically. Never let a player catch without the proper equipment. Keep up to date with the catcher's equipment, and always have good equipment on hand. The full equipment should be used even when the catcher is warming up.

Batter and Baserunner Equipment

A hard hat (batter's helmet) must be worn when batting. It should cover the temple and not be displaced when turning the head or running.

Uses of Protective Screens

The use of protective screens is necessary for productive practices. As these screens can be easily made in a metal shop, there is no excuse for not having them. Without such protection, the danger of catastrophic injury, including broken bones, paralysis, blindness, coma, and even death is increased.

There are several types of batting screens. These include a batting cage to cover the home plate area, a pitcher's protective screen, first and second base protective screens, and a batting practice ball shagger protective screen. These are discussed below.

Batting cage: The batting cage keeps all foul balls in the home plate area, and allows players or coaches to hit fungos to infielders from an area close to homeplate for full utilization of the diamond. There are many models to choose from, but the portable screen with wheels is the easiest to use.

Pitcher's protective screen: There are three basic shapes for the pitcher's protective screen. These are discussed briefly below:

1. Model 1 is an approximately four feet by four feet screen which protects the pitcher's lower body. The screen should be covered with 36 weight web, cyclone fencing, or anything functional and protective. This screen is not as protective as the other two, and is very hard to coach from behind.

2. Model 2 is L-shaped with the two outside dimensions eight feet, and all other dimensions four feet. This is basically the four feet

by four feet screen (Model 1) with a vertical four by eight section added. The lower section protects the pitcher's lower body; following the pitch the pitcher steps behind the upright section for full protection. This screen can be reversed for right- and left-handed pitchers.

3. Model 3 takes the idea further. There are half screens on both sides of the vertical so that no movement of the screen is necessary when switching from right- to left-handed pitchers.

Infielder's protective screen: All infield screens can be of standard size and will protect the first baseplayer, second base, and the ball shagger. Dimensions are approximately eight feet wide and nine feet high. The first base screen should be positioned about 10 feet in front of the base and on the first base foul line so that the first base player can still catch throws from third base. The second base screen should also be about 10 feet from the base, directly between the base and homeplate. The shagging screens should be about 10 feet onto the outfield grass and positioned to both sides of second base so that the center fielder can see the ball off the bat.

Coaching points: Never start an organized practice without the screens in position for player protection. Alert players of balls flying all over even though the screens are present.

6

Basketball

JON CHRISTOPHER
Washington State University
Pullman, Washington

POSSIBLE CATASTROPHIC INJURIES

Coaches need to inform their players of the following possible catastrophic injuries: 1) death, 2) loss of sight, 3) paraplegia, 4) quadriplegia, and 5) coma, with varying degrees of paralysis (Table 6-1).

PREVENTION OF CATASTROPHIC INJURIES

Warning of Dangers

Coaches must make their players aware that the primary cause of potential catastrophic injury involves violent or savage contact. Players must be informed that the following actions must not occur: excessive swinging of arms and elbows, striking with the fist or elbow, kicking, kneeing, running under a player who is in the air, or crouching or hipping in a manner which might cause a catastrophic injury to an opponent.

Coaches need to be aware that fatigue increases the potential for injury. Players exhibiting signs of fatigue should be removed from possible dangerous practice and game situations. Coaches should also inform their players that when they are fatigued they should ask to be replaced in order to recuperate.

Coaches need to make their players aware of any immovable objects within 10 feet of the playing court which, if struck, could result in a catastrophic injury. If the objects within this space are movable and are not required for the conduct of the game, they should be removed. Coaches must instruct players as to the potential danger involved in

Table 6-1. Possible Catastrophic Injuries in Basketball

Activity	Possible Injury	Causes	Prevention
Layup and dunk shot, Fast break	Paraplegia, Quadriplegia, Coma, Death	Undercutting, Shoving, Hipping	Proper instruction and practice drills on: 1) how to defend against person in the air, 2) catching themselves or opponents in a breakaway layup
Rebounding	Loss of sight, Coma, Death	Swinging elbows, Striking with fist	Proper instruction and insistence upon: 1) no swinging of elbows, 2) no striking with fist or violent behavior. Instruction and practice on how to properly rebound
Drills	Paraplegia, Quadriplegia, Loss of sight, Coma, Death	Collisions, Falls, Struck by thrown ball	Construct drills in an organizational pattern where one player or a thrown ball cannot cause injury to another player
Floor maintenance	Paraplegia, Quadriplegia, Coma	Falls	Continual care and upkeep of gym floor

grabbing the rim and also the danger involved in a dunk shot. Uncontrolled falls to the head, neck, or back can occur.

Proper Instruction and Correct Technique

Coaches must instruct players how to catch themselves or their opponents when they are placed in a body position that could cause possible injury. The greatest potential for catastrophic injury in basketball is cutting the legs out from under a player in the air. Players need to be informed of the proper method of taking a charging foul. A player taking a charging foul of an opponent who is in the air must remain stationary and not bend over, but should, with elbows hinged, place his or her hands between himself or herself and the opponent to help cushion the blow and to help catch the opponent. When an opponent has broken away for a layup and the player plans on committing a foul to prevent the opponent from making the layup, the player should never shove, but should grab and securely hold up the opponent. Once the opponent is in the air to shoot the layup, the player should not intentionally foul the shooter.

In rebounding or protecting the ball from the opponent, players should be instructed to broaden their base by spreading their feet slightly wider than shoulder width apart. Their arms should be about shoulder height with their elbows away from their bodies. The ball is protected by using the proper pivot to clear themselves from their opponents. Coaches must instruct their players they are never to swing their elbows in trying to protect the ball.

Coaches must construct drills so the drills will not be performed in organizational patterns where a player or a thrown ball can cause catastrophic injury to another player.

SPECIAL SAFETY CONSIDERATIONS

Rules

For the purpose of preventing catastrophic injuries, rules regarding improper player conduct have been very specifically identified with severe penalties for violations. Coaches need to know these rules and communicate clearly to their players that such rules are not to be violated.

Fouls—Flagrant: A flagrant foul may be personal or technical. It is always unsportsmanlike and may or may not be intentional. If personal, it involves violent or savage contact, such as striking with the fist or elbow, kicking, kneeing, running under a player who is in the air, or crouching or hipping in a manner which might cause severe injury to the opponent.

Excessive Swinging of Arms and Elbows: The current rules make it a violation for a player to excessively swing his or her arms or elbows when no opponent is contacted, and a foul if there is any contact. Special attention has now been given to these actions because they: 1) have resulted in injury to players, and 2) have placed opponents at a disadvantage, since defensive players could approach the offender only at the risk of suffering head or body injuries. Usually, this excessive swinging occurs following the recovery of a rebound, although the rules now consider such action illegal on all areas of the floor and under all circumstances.

With dunking made legal beginning with the 1976–77 season, rules were initiated because of the potential injury and damage to equipment factor. Grabbing the rim while dunking is a technical foul because of the possibility of causing a glass backboard to shatter with possible serious eye or head injuries. Collapsable rims are recommended and should be used.

Facilities and Equipment

With player safety a primary concern, the official rule book states that an official playing court shall have at least three feet (and preferably 10 feet) of unobstructed space outside. If, on an unofficial court, there are less than three feet of unobstructed space outside any sideline or endline, a narrow broken line shall be marked in the court parallel with and three feet inside that boundary. In general, court specifications should include dimensions as stated in basketball rules, ample out of bounds area, a id adequate seating space.

Padding for backboards: The following specifications should be adhered to for padding for the bottom and sides of the rectangular backboards:

1. The material must be rubber or plastic shock-absorbing material of the type approved for automobile dash boards.
2. The padding must cover the bottom surface of the board and the side surface to a distance of 15 inches up from the bottom.
3. The front surface must be covered to a minimum distance of three-fourths of an inch from the front edge.
4. The material shall not be less than two inches in thickness.
5. For uniformity, the padding shall be gray in color.
6. The committee recommends that the padding be mounted on the board by adhesive material.

Appropriate padding must also be used on any goal supports or any other objects within three feet unobstructed space outside the playing court. Recognizing that the official rule book identifies a preferred distance of 10 feet of unobstructed space outside the playing court, it is recommended that appropriate padding be used on objects within this space.

Prior to 1966–67, the rules, via the referee, did not permit any player to wear equipment considered dangerous to other players. This coverage was inadequate because some referees permitted certain types of equipment while other referees disallowed them. Because the referee was required to make the judgment, it was not uncommon for a player or coach to make a plea to the referee for permission to wear equipment that could be hazardous to the opposing team. The coverage was found wanting in some circumstances because it was not sufficiently specific. Rules had always prohibited the wearing of equipment which had a cutting edge or which could easily cause an abrasion. It was not considered in the spirit of the game then, nor is it today, to permit a player to wear a piece of equipment that will assist him in making contact with an opponent or protect the wearer from the impact of contact. The intent of the rules is to have players use only equipment which is specifically made for use in basketball.

The present rule lists several items which are always illegal even though they may be covered with soft padding. The 1976–77 season rule stated that elbow, hand, finger, wrist, or forearm guards, or casts or braces made of sole leather, plaster, pliable (soft) plastic, metal or any other hard substance, even though covered with soft padding, shall always be declared illegal. The change in this ruling is that the word "fore" has been added to the word "arm." The rule will now be slightly less restricted than it was in 1975–76, when it prohibited any such material to be on the arm at any point. Materials on the upper arm were not restricted beginning in 1976–77 provided, of course, they were covered with a soft foam rubber or equally soft protective covering. For example, a shoulder apparatus and chain might be extended around a player's upper arm and body to keep his shoulder from going out of joint due to a previous injury. Such protective equipment, if properly covered with soft material, will now be legal.

Coaches must periodically inspect their playing areas making sure that immovable objects required for the conduct of the game are properly padded and all other objects are removed in accordance with specifications of an official playing court. Records should be maintained noting the date of inspection and maintenance and repairs made. Proper cleaning of the gym floor must be maintained to prevent unnecessary falls in which the head or neck could be injured. Coaches should periodically check the shoe surface traction of their players to avert unnecessary falls. Perspiration may be deposited on the floor, causing players to slip if the moisture is not wiped away. Records of player injuries should be kept indicating date of injury, and medical treatment received. Coaches need to inspect the playing areas at "away games" and inform their players of any safety concerns. Coaches must refuse to play on unsafe courts.

7

Competitive Diving and Swimming

GERALD DEMERS
Washington State University
Pullman, Washington

Diving is a skill that involves many intricate motor patterns. Whether diving from the side of a pool, a starting block in competitive swimming, or the diving board, a diver must be aware of the potential hazards associated with the skill.

There are an estimated 8,000 to 9,000 diving related injuries each year sufficiently serious to be brought to hospital emergency wards (Gabrielsen 1981). Many of these injuries result in neck trauma which often leads to paralysis. Catastrophic, paralyzing spinal injuries occur in the United States each year at the rate of 30 to 35 per million population. This leads to approximately 7,700 new spinal injuries each year. Nearly 11 percent of these spinal injuries involve diving. Thus, about 800 spinal cord injuries result each year from diving into water areas such as swimming pools, lakes, ocean surf, and rivers. About half are due to persons diving into unsupervised areas from the banks of rivers, quarry ledges, boats, docks, and even trees (Gabrielsen 1981).

The trauma involved with neck injuries and the astronomical costs incurred by the individual and society necessitates a unified effort by all agencies involved with swimming and diving to identify and deal with this problem. The purpose of this chapter is to identify the potential hazards inherent in diving and swimming and offer ideas that will help reduce these potential risk factors.

Diving injuries related to swimming pool accidents can be divided into two categories: 1)springboard diving accidents; and 2)diving into shallow water. Since each constitutes a unique hazard, each will be dealt with separately. However, before discussing either circumstance, statistical data will be provided to help the reader understand the existing hazards involved with diving.

Several studies have been conducted on diving accidents. The University of Miami Medical School in conjunction with Nova University submitted a summary of *The Study of Medical Analysis of Selected Swimming Pool Injuries* to the Consumer Products Safety Commission. The main focus of the study was to investigate injuries occurring in swimming pools and to provide insight into the mechanism and severity of these accidents. Many of the following statistical references will relate to this study. Herein, information gathered from this study will be cited as (CPSC 1977).

An analysis of the swimming pool accidents studied indicated that in every instance the injuries occurred as a result of the victim striking the head on the bottom. All victims sustained spinal cord injuries of sufficient magnitude to render them quadriplegics. Some were extension type fractures, some flexion. Almost all of them also included compression type fractures. Most of the injuries occurred at the fourth, fifth, or sixth cervical vertebrae.

Gabrielsen (1980) related that the number of quadriplegic injuries resulting from diving exceeded by a wide margin the total from all other sports combined—football, water skiing, gymnastics, track, trampoline, wrestling, snow skiing, and surfing. He assisted in compiling data from 75 swimming pool accident cases, in addition to the results of the CPSC medical study. This provided a total of 132 accident cases, all resulting in injury to the spinal cord, with 122 resulting in quadriplegia. Of these injuries, 31 resulted from diving from a diving board and 62 resulted from diving into shallow water. Tables 7-1 and 7-2 present summaries of where and how these accidents occurred.

Table 7-1. Accidents While Diving from Springboards or Jumpboards

A.	Three-meter high boards	8
B.	One-meter high boards	3
C.	Springboards 12 feet or less in length or jumpboards	20
		31

Table 7-2. Accidents While Diving into Shallow Portion of Pool

A.	From the deck of inground pools into water four feet deep or less	34
B.	Platforms, deck, or coping of above ground pools	15
C.	Dive into shallow portion of pool toward hopper	6
D.	Ladder attached to above ground pools	5
E.	Starting blocks used for competition	2
		62

From the information previously listed and a more thorough review of the results of the studies cited, it can be surmised that certain factors or conditions have a greater influence on possible injury than others. In the use of springboards, insufficient water depth in the diving area was a major contributing factor to spinal injuries. Insufficient bottom markings and slippery surfaces on the bottom are other contributory factors. Diving into shallow water is the major contributing cause of serious neck injuries. Factors that contributed to many of these injuries include: inadequate water depth, lack of bottom markings, size of victims, absence of warnings, and absence of depth markings.

It was observed that some of the victims displayed poor judgment in diving into shallow water. However, there is great significance in the fact that a large percentage of the victims had been in the pool of question on three or less occasions (CPSC 1977). Another general conclusion is that certain pool designs have definite limitations with regard to the kinds of activities that can safely be conducted in them. Bottom angles, hopper bottom pools, and vertical walls present many of these limitations.

Now that many of the hazards have been identified, it is important that steps be taken to eliminate potential risk factors and conduct proper instructional progressions to avoid accidents. The remaining information in this chapter will deal with preventive teaching techniques and proper handling of neck injuries.

SPRINGBOARD DIVING

The untrained diver is the most likely candidate for a neck injury. Generally, the neophyte diver makes a water entry with the hands and arms over head. After making contact with the surface of the water the arms collapse which exposes the head for contact with any obstruction.

Many people have a misconception that it takes a high degree of velocity to sustain a neck injury. Biomechanical studies indicate neck injuries can occur with head impact velocities in the range of eight to 10 feet per second. Velocities of more than 20 feet per second are easily attained in free standing dives (CPSC 1977).

Striking the bottom with the head in a flexed position fixes the head for the impacting weight of the diver's following body. Only a slight blow to the head in such a position is required to cause the flexion type fracture in the C-5 or C-6 region of the spine (Gabrielsen 1981). In springboard diving, divers are taught to hold the arms over the head, align the arms with the body and tighten the muscles upon entry into the water. All of these methods, combined with the spring and lift into the air, as well as a near vertical entry, contribute to the velocity of the diver under water. This velocity would be sufficient to cause a severe neck injury if the diver's head hit the bottom of the pool.

Accident Prevention and Proper Instruction

It was previously mentioned that the leading cause of neck injuries in diving was hitting the head on the bottom of a shallow pool. Therefore, it is important for the instructor or coach to teach the correct methods for safe water entries.

At this time it is important to note that in the literature reviewed (CPSC 1977; Gabrielsen 1981), none of the accidents reported occurred in pools meeting the recommended dimensions for diving facilities suggested by the National Collegiate Athletic Association (NCAA), United States Diving (USD), or FINA (the international governing body for aquatics).

Unfortunately, not all pools meet these specifications, which may present some hazards. The following is a list of possible hazards a competitive diver may encounter while diving in competition at home or away.

Hazard Number 1: Water Depth

One major hazard is diving into a pool where the water depth under the diving boards does not meet recommended standards. The recommended depth below a one-meter diving board is 11 feet (USD, FINA), while the depth below a three-meter diving board should be at least 12 feet (USD, FINA). The recommended minimum depth for a 10-meter platform diving area is 18 feet. However, when a water entry is executed with a minimum of drag, a competitive diver will contact the bottom at an extremely high velocity even at these recommended depths. Therefore, it is important for the competitive diver to maintain the hands over the head for impact with the bottom.

Another hazard is competing in pools where the deep water is shallower than the deep water in which the competitive diver practices. A diver becomes accustomed to a certain depth and the timing relative to impact with the bottom. It is, therefore, important to note the depth of the pool and bottom configurations to prepare for a change in that timing. The biggest problem is adjusting the timing to shallower pools. Impact with the bottom is quicker, and the diver must be prepared.

Prevention

The coach should inform divers of any difference in bottom depth. A progression can then be implemented to help each diver acclimate to the different conditions. The following progression will help divers safely adjust to the unfamiliar pool depth.

1. Diver identifies depth markings.
2. Diver submerges with goggles or mask and checks bottom contours.
3. Diver jumps from the end of the one-meter diving board feet first

and keeps the body streamlined and rigid. This allows the diver to develop a sense of timing while hitting the bottom feet first.

4. Diver does a head first dive while standing on the end of the diving board, maintaining the hands and arms over the head.
5. Diver does a head first dive with an approach.

The head first dive should be a simple dive, such as a front dive in the tuck position. This will allow the diver to concentrate on the entry and the timing of impact with the bottom. Each step in the progression should be repeated several times for optimal safety. This same progression should also be used from the three-meter diving board.

Hazard Number 2: Bottom Configurations

Not all pools are designed the same way. There are variations in bottom contours that may present a hazard. The ideal pool bottom for springboard diving is one in which the bottom in the diving area is flat. Many pools have slopes in the bottom contour that begin in the diving area. One of the most hazardous contours is one in which the deepest point in the pool is located at the intersection of a "V" bottom contour.

In a pool such as this, the depth marking located on the deck generally indicates the deepest point. On many occasions, the diver will not contact the bottom at the deepest point in the pool. Depending on the point of contact with the bottom, the diver may encounter an equivalent of a one- to two-foot variation in depth. Backward approaches seem to cause the biggest problem. Back and inward dives may end up in shallower water because of the underwater trajectory of the diver.

Prevention

The coach should emphasize the hazard of the bottom contour to the divers and point out the probability of making contact with the bottom sooner than expected. An underwater save (breakdown of the streamlined body position underwater) will create more drag and slow the velocity of the diver. This skill should be taught by all coaches and practiced to the point of mastery by all divers.

Other potential hazards due to bottom contours should also be pointed out by the coach. Additional bottom configurations that may present a hazard include:

1. Safety ledge underneath the diving board. This produces a shorter distance from the plummet (end of the diving board) to the wall underneath the diving board.
2. Hopper Bottoms, which greatly reduce the deep areas underneath the diving boards.
3. Pools with restricted deep water surface areas for divers to land.
4. Bottom incline slopes that are too steep in gradient and too close to the diving area.

5. Abrupt walls in diving wells. These walls may be located too close to the plummet, out in front of the diving board.

All pool bottom contours that present a hazard should be clearly marked. Black diagonal stripes on the bottom, inclines, or vertical obstructions will help the unsuspecting diver identify the hazards.

Hazard Number 3: Slippery Pool Bottoms and Diving Boards

Slippery pool bottoms are the cause of several neck injuries per year; these injuries occur in pools with a variety of bottom surfaces. If pool chemistry is not maintained properly, algae may accumulate on the bottom, creating an extremely slippery surface. If a diver hits the bottom of the pool where algae has grown, the diver's hands may slip out of line, which will expose the head for impact with the bottom.

Prevention

Preventive maintenance is the best method of curing algae problems. This can be accomplished by maintaining high levels of free available chlorine with periodic superchlorination [Washington State Public Health Association (WSPHA) n.d.]. Various forms of algicides can also be added to the water to help reduce or prevent algae growth. Quaternary ammonia compounds are also effective in combating algae; however, there may be eye irritation due to the chlormines that are formed during use of these compounds (WSPHA n.d.).

Diving boards are susceptible to algae growth also. Along with the algae growth, the rough surface of the diving board seems to retain body oils and other body lotions. These oils, combined with dust particles, can create a slippery surface in a relatively short period of time.

Prevention

Once again, proper maintenance is the solution to this problem. Diving boards should be cleaned with a high-pressure sprayer at least three times a week in an indoor pool and more often in outdoor pools because of the dust accumulation. A short-term solution to this problem, if confronted with a slippery board at a facility other than the one in which practice is held, is to spray the board surface and apply a solution of 12 percent sodium hypochlorite (liquid chlorine) or calcium hypochlorite (granular chlorine). Allow this to set for 15 minutes and then hose off thoroughly.

Hazard Number 4: Diver Making Contact With the Diving Board

While catastrophic neck injuries resulting from divers hitting diving boards are rare, these devastating injuries are recognized hazards in the sport of diving. Diving requires a high degree of skill in order to execute the variety of dives performed in competition. Even the highly skilled, expertly trained divers, on occasion, flirt with disaster due to a lapse in concentration or mistake in execution of a dive. Although it is not a very pleasant task to discuss these injuries, it is a reality of the sport. The dives that seem to create the highest incidence of injury due to contact with the diving board include inward dives, reverse dives, and reverse twisting dives.

The inward group of dives consists of a backward take-off followed by a rotating motion toward the diving board. The inward somersaulting action adds velocity to the rotation, and if contact is made with the diving board, a neck injury could result. If the head contacts the board, a flexion or flexion-compression neck injury may occur. It is also possible to sustain an extension injury.

The reverse dive and reverse somersaulting dive may also result in a head or neck injury if contact is made with the diving board. If the reverse dive is not performed at a proper distance from the diving board the diver may hit the diving board resulting in an extension, extension-compression, compression, flexion-compression, or flexion fracture. The same types of fractures may occur during reverse rotating dives.

Reverse twisting dives present a unique problem, because at the completion of the twisting action, the diver bends at the waist and looks toward the water. In this dive, the diver executes a forward approach and initiates a somersaulting action rotating backward. The twist action is completed with the diver facing the diving board. If the diver executes the take-off improperly, the end result may put the diver in the air directly above the diving board. During head-first entries, the head may be exposed to impact with the diving board resulting in a neck injury.

Prevention

Although the diver may make contact with the board on a number of different dives, the aforementioned dives seem to present a greater possibility of a catastrophic injury. Prevention of this type of injury is best accomplished by utilizing proper teaching progressions and having a thorough knowledge of physical laws as they relate to diving. There are several books relative to springboard diving that present many safe progressions to follow during the learning phase. *The Techniques of Springboard Diving*, by Charles Batterman (1968), is, in this author's opinion, the best book available relative to physical laws in springboard diving. If the coach utilizes the proper progressions, the safety of the diver will be greatly enhanced.

Unfortunately, accidents occur even if the proper progressions are taught. Maintaining an environment that eliminates outside disturbances will aid the diver in concentration. Maintaining diving equipment will also reduce the possibility of an accident. Diving boards should be level. Any upward pitch will result in a diver being catapulted toward the diving board. The greater the angle of the pitch, the more likely the diver will be in close proximity to the diving board.

Hazard Number 5: "Rip Entry" Technique

An entry technique that reduces the amount of splash is being taught and used throughout the world. The term most often used for this new technique is "Rip Entry," because of the unique sound that is created if the entry is successful. The sound is similar to that made when tearing a piece of cloth. When mastered, this entry produces no splash and leaves the judges with an impression of "extraordinary execution" of the dive. When executing this entry, the diver pulls the arms laterally toward the sides upon contact with the water. This action exposes the head and may result in the head hitting the bottom of the pool. If the pool is deep enough, the diver will have enough time to recover the arms back into position over the head before making contact with the bottom. A POOL DEPTH OF 16 FEET OR DEEPER IS NEEDED TO SAFELY PERFORM THE RECOVERY. The alternative is to alter the body position to avoid contact with the bottom. Altering the body position, as in performing a "save," creates drag and slows the descent or redirects the trajectory of the diver underwater. The point to remember is that even if a save is executed, the head is still exposed. A high degree of skill is needed in order to avoid an injury in this circumstance.

Prevention

The greatest preventive measure is the responsibility of the coach. The coach must employ a sequence of proper progressions in order to develop the skill necessary to avoid injury. First of all, the novice competitive diver should be taught proper body alignment for entries. The arms and hands should remain over the head during these entries. The next step would be to teach the diver how to "save" a dive. These skills are more advanced, and it may take a great deal of time to develop the techniques. A diver should know how to perform a properly aligned entry before "saves" are taught. After the diver has mastered the art of "saving" a dive, the coach can then teach the procedures and techniques utilized for "Rip Entries."

Progressions for safely teaching the "Rip Entry:"

1. From the side of the pool in deep water, practice the arm and body motions involved in this type of entry. If pike saves are used, the diver must jump far enough from the side to avoid hitting the head on the side of the pool.
2. From the end of the diving board, dive into the water with moderate spring and perform the "Rip Entry."
3. From the diving board, use a forward approach and perform a front dive tuck and "Rip Entry" (the diver can concentrate on the entry and not have to worry about the execution of the dive).
4. From the diving board use a forward approach, execute any given dive, and perform the "Rip Entry."

These progressions should also be used off the three-meter diving board. Water depth should be 16 feet or deeper if a save is not used. After the diver has mastered these techniques, there may still be some hazards. Once again, when diving in an unfamiliar pool it is extremely important to identify the pool depth in the diving area, the bottom contour, and the length of the landing area. If the water is shallower than that to which the diver is accustomed, it may be wise to cancel the use of the "Rip Entry" techniques. This is a judgment decision which should be carefully considered and made prior to the practice or competition. The welfare of the diver is at stake, and the risk may be extensive.

The sport of diving can be made safer by identifying the hazards in your home pool and pools one may visit during competition. Make your pool a safer place to dive by clearly posting depth markings and diving rules, maintaining proper pool chemistry, clearly marking the bottom, marking potential hazards due to bottom contour, and utilizing proper teaching progression. If this can be done effectively, divers, coaches, and parents will appreciate the concern for safety in the sport.

DIVING INTO SHALLOW WATER (COMPETITIVE RACING STARTS)

When one considers risk factors relative to competitive swimming, it is difficult to imagine catastrophic injuries occurring in this sport. However, diving once again is the hazard. The start of a race is generally conducted in shallow water. Most competitive pools range from three-and-one-half feet to four feet in depth in the shallow section. Racing starts, if performed incorrectly, could result in a neck injury with possible paralysis. Striking the bottom of the pool during a racing dive is a possibility, and the coach should keep this in mind when teaching the various techniques incorporated in racing starts.

If the swimmer enters the water "cleanly" (has the long axis of the body aligned with the direction of entry), the drag of the water has a negligible effect upon the swimmer's velocity until he or she is almost fully immersed. Therefore, diving at angles greater than 30 degrees into shallow water (less than five feet) can lead to the head striking the bottom at potentially dangerous velocities.

The height of the diver is an important factor. The taller diver requires deeper water for an acceptable safety level. The weight of the diver does not influence the velocities to any great extent, but may well contribute to a neck injury. In a diving accident with resulting neck injury, the head invariably strikes something. If the head impact occurs against the pool bottom, the diver's body will continue moving, either flexing or extending the neck, depending on the attitude of the body at impact. This results in a folding action with the potential to cause severe dislocation. The heavier the torso, the more severe is the neck loading in this case (CPSC 1977). With the emphasis that is being placed on "streamlining" (maintaining body alignment in the water), drag is greatly reduced, increasing initial velocities in the water on a racing start and maintaining greater velocities for longer distances under water.

There are a number of techniques that have been adopted in recent years to help the swimmer reduce drag and increase distance and velocity in racing starts. Most of these techniques result in the swimmer staying fairly close to the surface upon water entry. If these techniques are used, it is still critical to stress the importance of maintaining the arms over the head for protection.

Hazard Number 1: "Dive-In-The-Hole" Racing Start

Coaches are always investigating new methods for racing starts that will give their athletes an edge over the competition. Recently, a new technique for racing starts, called the "Dive-In-The-Hole," has been incorporated into most competitive programs throughout the world. Without going into any great detail about the technique, basically the dive is designed to maximize underwater velocity by reducing hydrodynamic drag. In this particular start the swimmer's body travels in an arc rather than a flattened path. At the peak of this arc the swimmer pikes at the hips, which lowers the head and arms in preparation for the water entry. This technique creates less drag in the water because the entire body will enter close to the same point where the hands enter. The swimmer, in effect, creates a hole with the hands and the body enters through that hole. If this technique is performed correctly, the swimmer will enter the water at a 30- to 40-degree angle (Maglischo 1982). Some coaches advocate a steeper angle of entry. This is where the hazard exists. The swimmer must immediately redirect the hands and head towards the surface in an arching motion in order to avoid collision with the pool bottom.

The Consumer Product Safety Commission (1977) reported that the path or trajectory of a diver will vary in accordance with the action of the arms and legs, the body's starting position, and the lean of the body at the takeoff. The strong athletic type can spring forward to easily enter the water at a spot nine or 10 feet from the edge of the pool. The path the diver's body takes cannot be changed appreciably by the diver once in the air. The action that is potentially most dangerous when the dive is made in shallow water is breaking sharply at the hips, which places the diver in a semijackknife position. When the diver's angle at entry is 30 degrees or less and the diver proceeds to drop the arms and head, the body will be placed in an angle from 45 degrees to 90 degrees (vertical entry). This will place the diver on a collision course with the bottom, even in depths of eight or nine feet, if the body alignment is maintained. When a swimmer enters at an angle in excess of 45 degrees in shallow water (three to five feet), there is practically no time to arch and change direction back toward the surface.

This skill is difficult to master even for an accomplished competitive swimmer, yet younger children are being taught this method to improve their performance standards. It is extremely important that the coach recognize this potential hazard and guard against placing any competitive swimmer in jeopardy of a neck injury.

Prevention

Although there are risks involved with performing this start, it is an effective method for increasing distance during the start of a competitive event. As long as the technique is effective, coaches will continue to use this method until a new and better technique is devised. If a coach decides to teach this technique to the competitive swimmer, it should be noted that there are potential risks involved. The coach should seriously consider the athletic ability of each swimmer who will be taught this skill. If there is any doubt as to the ability of the swimmer to perform this style of racing start, the coach should reconsider presenting the technique to such an individual.

Due to injuries that have occurred and multi-million dollar lawsuits that have resulted from performance of this racing start, this skill should *NOT* be used where water depth is five feet or less.

If the proper progressions are used when teaching this skill the coach can greatly reduce the potential of an injury. The following are steps in a progression that should be adopted for teaching the "Dive-In-The-Hole" racing start:

1. The first consideration should be the arm position over the head. It should be emphasized that the arms should remain in position over the head at least until the swimmer begins to return to the surface. The arms will aid in protecting the head if the swimmer makes contact with the bottom inadvertently.
2. Since this skill involves a dive at an angle greater than 30 degrees, the next progression should consist of a series of repetitions from the *side* of the swimming pool in *deep* water (10 to 12 feet deep). The mechanics of the start can be learned in this safer environment which will lower the risk factors. Mistakes in technique will not result in a collision with the bottom. If underwater windows are available, the coach can observe the technique underwater and determine if the dive is safe. If underwater windows are not available, a face mask can be used. Markings placed on the wall in the deep water to indicate four feet and five feet depths will aid the coach in determining if the depth of the racing dive will be hazardous if attempted in shallower water.
3. After completing a series of dives from the side of the pool, the dive should be done from a starting block in deep water. The

swimmer will reach a greater height in the arc of the dive and therefore will have a greater velocity upon entry into the water. There is also an increased probability of entering the water at a greater angle. Diving from the starting blocks in deep water enables the swimmer to develop the timing and coordination needed to safely complete the start from a greater height. Once again, the coach should observe the dive from underwater to determine if the depth the swimmer achieves is safe.

4. After mastering the technique in deep water, the next step is to attempt the dive in shallower water (five to six feet deep). The same procedures should be followed in this depth as was mentioned in B and C above. A series of dives should be attempted in order to determine the safety of the skill being performed. This type of racing start should be attempted only by experienced competitive swimmers.

Although these progressions will help the swimmer develop the necessary skills to safely perform the Dive-In-The-Hole racing start, other safety precautions can be implemented to minimize the risk. The following are suggestions to reduce the potential hazards:

1. Secure all starting blocks at the deep end of the pool.
2. Depth markings should be placed on the deck near the edge of the pool and on the interior wall above the water line. These markings should be in a contrasting color and should be at least four inches high (six inches preferred). Depth markings indicating separation of deep water from shallow water must be located exactly at the breakpoint and must coincide with the exact depth (CNCA 1975).
3. Make sure the bottom has clear markings to aid the swimmer in determining depth and location of the bottom.
4. Do not allow a swimmer to attempt this start if there is any doubt concerning the individual's ability to perform the skill safely.
5. If your pool is too shallow for this type of start, have the competitors on all teams utilize the flat racing start in competition. Warn visiting teams of the possible hazards by letter and verbally before the competition.

Hazard Number 2: Impact With the Side of the Pool

Another potential catastrophic injury may result from impact with the head on the side of the pool. Although this is not common in strokes performed in the prone position, it may happen while a swimmer is executing the back crawl. A competitive swimmer can generate enough force during the back crawl to cause a compression or compression-flexion type of neck injury. Upon impact, the head remains relatively in place, while the torso continues to move toward the head. The force created by the impact combined with the weight of the body driving toward the head could cause substantial damage.

Prevention

Backstroke flags should be in position at all times while swimmers are practicing backstroke turns or the backstroke. Practice the timing for the turns at your home pool and at competitions in other pools. Make sure the backstroke flag specifications are met (consult the appropriate rule book). Lane-lines should have contrasting colors the last 15 feet on each end.

Hazard Number 3: Concurrent Swimming and Diving Team Practice Schedule

In competitive programs where diving and swimming teams practice concurrently in a pool without a diving well, there is a potential hazard of a diver landing on a swimmer. This creates the risk of injury to the swimmer and diver. On a head first entry the diver may injure the neck. There may be other minor injuries to both the swimmer and the diver. If the diver lands on the back of a swimmer, there is a possibility of a broken back.

Prevention

Although there are benefits with respect to maintaining team cohesion by conducting concurrent practices, safety must be a consideration. Different practice times for swimmers and divers eliminates the hazard completely. If this is not possible, use lane-lines to divide the pool to allow a safe diving area without swimmers. If this procedure is followed it is important to locate the lane-lines at a safe distance to the side of the line of flight of the diver. If the lane-lines are too close to the diving board, a new hazard has been produced.

If correct preventive measures are established, the swimming and diving program will flourish with reduced risk of injury. The coach should take the responsibility to administer a program that will insure the welfare of every competitor.

CARE OF NECK INJURIES IN AN AQUATIC ENVIRONMENT

If a neck injury occurs in your swimming pool, it is extremely important that necessary equipment is readily available. It is also important that the coach know how to implement an effective rescue. The CPSC (1977) observed that in only 13 of the 72 cases they studied were proper rescue procedures employed. It is highly likely that a significant portion of the persons suffering spinal cord injuries have further loss of neurological function and exacerbation of their deficits by mishandling at the accident scene. It is the intent of this section to list the equipment that should be readily available and introduce effective procedures for handling neck injuries.

Equipment

The following equipment should be readily available for use in case of a possible neck injury:

1. Spine board—located on the pool deck: should have a sufficient number of straps to immobilize the head, chest, hips, legs, and feet.
2. Sand bags—used to stabilize the head once the victim is placed on the spine board.
3. First Aid Kit—located in the pool office.
4. Telephone—located in the pool office or on the pool deck. Emergency phone numbers should be attached to the phone.
5. Blankets—located in the pool office.

Handling Potential Neck Injuries

If the victim was performing a skill that presented a possible neck injury, handle it as such. The manner in which the victim is handled may add insult to injury or prevent further damage. There are a number of methods that have been devised for handling neck injuries in the water.

The American Red Cross (1973) presents the following method:

> If the victim is floating face down, turn him over carefully with the least amount of movement, keeping his head and body aligned. Place one of your hands in the middle of the victim's back with your arm right over his head; place your other hand under the victim's upper arm close to the shoulder, ready to run him to the face up position. Rotate the victim by lifting his shoulder up and over with one hand while your other hand and arm support and maintain his head and body alignment.

In a procedure discussed by Davis and McFeters (1974), it was emphasized that the victim's head should always be kept in line with the body and that the victim should be moved as one complete unit. They suggest that the victim should be sandwiched between the arms of the rescuer. One hand is placed on the back between the lower part of the shoulder blades with the fingers spread and somewhat parallel to the spine. The other hand is placed on the lower chest with the hand covering the lower half of the breastbone (sternum) with the fingers spread. The pressure of the two hands toward each other makes it possible to control the alignment of the victim's body. The rescuer should then start to back up while rolling the victim over. This motion will lift the legs toward the surface and therefore reduce lower back bend.

DeMers (1983) states that although there are procedures for rescuing a victim with a possible neck injury, the procedures currently used can be difficult to implement, especially when the victim is submerged in deep water. There are some important factors to consider when rescuing a victim with a possible neck injury. One of the most important factors is the stabilization of the victim's head and neck in the position in which they were found. Movement of the head or neck could cause further damage to the spinal column. A second factor to consider is the position of the victim's body before the rescue attempt. If the victim is face-down (prone) on the surface, he or she must be turned over to allow breathing. The rescuer must rotate the body to a face-up (supine) position without altering the head or neck position. A third factor to consider is submersion. If the victim is submerged, the rescuer must decide how to get him or her to the surface without altering the head and neck position. The final factor in a rescue attempt is the stabilization of the head and neck while on the surface or while towing the victim to shallow water before using a spine board. The following rescue procedure takes into consideration all of the aforementioned situations and presents an effective method of rescue.

Stabilization of the Head and Neck

The major objective of an effective rescue procedure involving a possible neck injury is to maintain the head and neck in the same position in which they were found when the victim was approached. Grasping both arms just above the elbows and moving them laterally upward so that the arms are extended on each side of the head, traps the head between the arms and provides a splint-like effect for stabilizing the head and neck (Figure 7-1). Moving the arms into this position will eliminate rotation, flexion, extension, and lateral movement of the head and neck if performed properly. To perform correctly, the rescuer must apply continuous pressure on the arms in order to hold the head in its original position (Figure 7-2). One concern involving this procedure was whether or not the movement of the arms would put undue stress on the cervical vertebrae. Five orthopedic surgeons and one neurosurgeon were consulted, and all concurred that such a movement would not affect the cervical vertebrae and would not put undue stress on the neck region. The following procedures are presented in relation to the position of the victim's body upon rescue.

Prone Position on the Surface:

Grasping the arms just above the elbows and moving the arms against the head will enable the rescuer to splint the head and neck in a stable position. Once secure, the rescuer should begin turning the victim into a supine position to enable the victim to breathe. The rescuer must apply pressure on the arms, inward, toward the head in order to maintain the head and neck position (Figure 7-3). The turning motion will slightly alter the position of the lower back, but if the victim's arms are kept stable there will be no change in the position of the head or neck (cervical vertebrae).

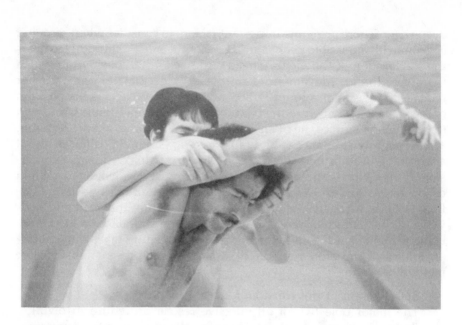

Figure 7-1. Arm position for head-splint procedure. Retrieval of victim from beneath the surface.

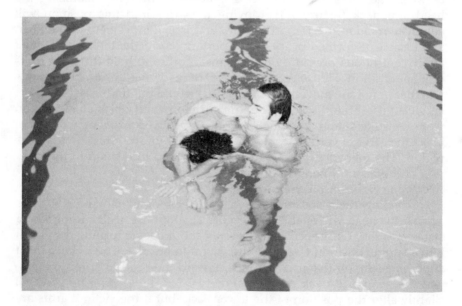

Figure 7-2. Head-splint procedure when the victim is in a prone position on the surface.

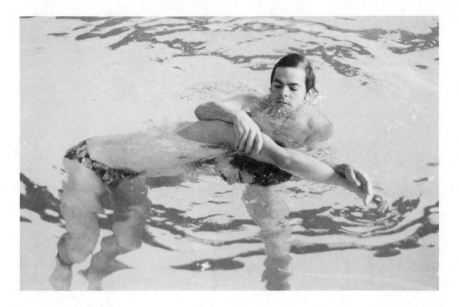

Figure 7-3. Turning the victim from a prone position to a supine position on the surface.

Supine Position on the Surface in Deep Water:
If the victim is found in a supine position on the surface, the rescuer should grasp the arms and move them laterally to apply the head-splint. The rescuer can then tow the victim to shallow water.

Underwater Retrieval:
Occasionally neck injuries may occur in deep water. If the victim remains under water, the rescuer can utilize the head-splint method to tow the victim to the surface. The arms should be moved slowly and laterally into a position in which the head can be stabilized. The rescuer should be positioned toward the rear of the victim which will enable the rescuer to pull the victim to the surface and more readily attain a supine position once at the surface (see Figure 7-1). When at the surface, the victim is in position to be towed to shallow water.

Towing the Victim
When in deep water, the head-splint method provides a stable easy method of transport. Once the victim is turned to a supine position on the surface, the rescuer should then begin towing the victim to the side of the pool or to shallow water where a spine board can be used (see Figure 7-4).

The head-splint rescue can be used in shallow water as well as deep water. It can also be effective in retrieving a victim from under water.

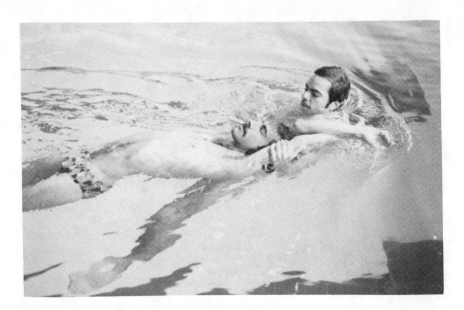

Figure 7-4. Towing the victim in deep water.

Aquatic related neck injuries occur in a variety of circumstances. The head-splint rescue procedure is a quick and effective method of rescue and can easily be adapted to all neck injuries in an aquatic environment. This rescue offers a method of stabilizing the head and neck effectively and is easy to apply.

Neck injuries in an aquatic environment may result from a variety of causes. Diving into shallow water or diving from a diving board represent the greatest hazards for the recreational and competitive swimmer or diver. Many neck injuries can be prevented if proper safety precautions and proper instructions are offered. The coach and athlete should become aware of the possible hazards in all swimming pools where they will be competing. Recognizing the hazards and improvising to eliminate the potential risks will enable the competitor to perform at minimal risk. Proper safety equipment should be immediately available, and all competitors, coaches, and lifeguards should know the correct techniques for rescuing a victim with a possible neck injury. Prevention of catastrophic neck injuries in competitive swimming or diving by insuring safety and using proper teaching progressions will contribute to the well-being of the participants in the sport.

8

Field Hockey

SANDRA MOORE
Kenyon College
Gambier, Ohio

The nature of the game of field hockey has changed rapidly in the past few years. Improved training programs, skill techniques, and strategies have combined to produce a faster game. The increased speed and the use of a hard ball and a stick, along with fast artificial turf playing fields, increase the potential for catastrophic injury (Table 8-1).

POSSIBLE CATASTROPHIC INJURIES

Potential serious injuries in hockey include:
1. A loss of vision caused by a blow to the eye by a stick or ball.
2. Brain damage resulting from a player being struck in the head by a stick or ball, or two players banging their heads together while attempting to play the same ball.

PREVENTION OF CATASTROPHIC INJURIES

All participants should be warned that:
1. A lack of proper conditioning can lead to fatigue, causing catastrophic injury.
2. Extended periods of physical activity, particularly in warm weather, result in loss of body fluids that must be replaced, or heat exhaustion may occur. Frequent water breaks are necessary.
3. The stick can cause serious injury if used improperly.
4. A blow to the head caused by a stick or ball could cause brain damage.
5. Permanent damage to the eye or loss of vision can occur if the ball or stick strikes the eye.

Table 8-1. Possible Catastrophic Injuries in Field Hockey

Skill	Injury	Cause	Proper Instruction	Safety Hints
Dribbling	Concussion, Loss of consciousness, Brain damage, Death	Banging of heads together	Keep ball well in front, bend knees, flex legs, and look up	Proper body control. Emphasize looking up. Include drills designed to improve body control and looking up while dribbling
Shot at goal	Concussion, Brain damage, Ruptured Spleen or other organs, Death	Fast driven ball hits goalkeeper	Player positioning for visibility. Protective equipment. Technique training in stopping drive at goal	Situational drills with successive shots at goalkeeper without other defensive players. Corner situational drills with complete defense
Drive	Loss of eye, Concussion, Loss of consciousness, Brain damage, Death	Raising of stick above shoulder height	Move stick back in a straight line until wrists are just below waist level. Cock wrists so head of stick is slightly above right hand. Keep wrists and grip firm. Tense shoulder, arm, wrist, and hand muscles at moment of contact. Follow through in the intended direction of the hit	Rule: A player shall not raise any part of his/her stick above the shoulder either at the beginning or at the end of a stroke when approaching, attempting to play, playing the ball, or stopping the ball. Don't allow high sticks. Don't allow balls in the air to be played with sticks
		Undercut ball	Keep weight forward. Keep head over ball. Transfer weight from rear to front	Rule: A player shall not hit wildly into an opponent or play the ball in such a way as to be dangerous itself or likely to lead to dangerous play. Emphasize: controlling a ball before attempting to hit it

Table 8-1. Continued

Skill	Injury	Cause	Proper Instruction	Safety Hints
Flick	Concussion, Loss of consciousness, Brain damage, Death	Hit in head with lofted ball	Combine transfer of body weight from rear to front foot with a forceful movement of the right forearm and strong wrist action in the direction of the pass. Keep the ball on the stick as long as possible in a throwing action	Rule: same as for an undercut ball. Guidance: a player should be penalized who by raising the ball is guilty of or directly causes dangerous play. Emphasize: flicks should be into a space, not people
Receiving	Concussion, Loss of consciousness, Brain damage, Death	Rebound off improperly fielded ball	Relax wrists and hands to absorb force of ball. Blade of stick at right angles to direction ball is coming from. Trap ball to avoid rebound in the air	Rule: same as for an undercut ball. Guidance: players should be penalized for dangerous play resulting from raising the ball in any way. A rising ball is dangerous when it causes legitimate evasive action on the part of the players. Emphasize: not hitting a ball before it is controlled; not fielding a ball that is hit in the air

CORRECT TECHNIQUES TO AVOID INJURY

Catastrophic injuries in field hockey are not common. However, the potential for serious injury exists and must be considered. Proper techniques in dribbling, receiving, driving, and flicking should be emphasized to reduce the risk of injury.

Dribbling

The stick is held with the left hand on top and the right hand about 10 inches down the handle. In a straight dribbling position, the back of the left hand faces upward, and the left wrist and forearm are a straight extension of the stick. The left elbow is well away from the body. The stick is held at a 45-degree angle to the ground, and the ball is played about 18 inches diagonally in front of the right foot. When dribbling, the legs are slightly flexed to allow the player to look up as forward progress is made.

In Indian dribbling, the same basic body position is taken while the stick is rotated over the ball so that contact is made with the flat side of the stick. The important point is that the ball is played well in front of the feet and the legs are flexed. This allows the player to look up to avert collisions and serious injury.

Receiving

Players need to be able to field balls approaching at varying speeds. The ball must be controlled to prevent it from rebounding dangerously in the air. The key to controlling the ball is the "giving" with the ball as it contacts the stick. This is accomplished by relaxing the tension of the grip (particularly of the right hand) as contact is made.

The grip and foot position vary as the ball is received from different angles. Regardless of the angle, important points to remember are that the eyes should be focused on the ball until it contacts the stick, the blade of the stick should be at a right angle or less to the direction from which the ball is coming, and the ball should be "trapped" to prevent upward deflection. Trapping is accomplished by inclining the blade of the stick toward the ground and the ball.

Driving

In the drive, the left hand is held at the top of the stick with the back of the hand facing the intended direction of the hit. The right hand is placed directly below and touching the left hand. The ball is about 18 inches in front of and opposite the heel of the left foot. The feet are shoulder width apart, and the left shoulder faces the direction of the pass.

The stick is pulled straight back with the left arm straight and the right elbow tucked into the side. When the wrists reach waist height, they cock so the head of the stick goes above the right wrist and the toe of the stick points upward but not higher than shoulder level. The wrists and grip remain firm.

The downswing is an acceleration of the stick in a straight line at the ball. At contact, the muscles of the shoulders, arms, wrists, and hands are firm. The arms are straight and follow through with the stick in the direction of the hit. The key point of emphasis for safety is that the wrists and grip remain firm. This allows the head of the stick to be controlled on the backswing and follow-through. The stroke should be kept below shoulder height.

Flicking

The grip for the flick is like the dribbling grip with the right hand a little further down on the stick. The body is turned sideways, with the left shoulder pointing in the intended direction of the ball. The feet are comfortably apart, and the ball is played off the left foot. The stick is placed under and behind the ball at a 45-degree angle to the ground. The shift of the body weight from the rear foot forward, coupled with a whipping action of the arms and wrists, gives impetus to the flick. The follow-through is a continuation of the whipping action through the ball.

For safety reasons, accuracy in this stroke is important. The player must be able to control the height and direction of the flick in order to avoid flicking the ball directly at an opponent. The whipping action and the follow-through are important factors in keeping the head of the stick safely below shoulder height.

PROGRESSION OF SKILL DEVELOPMENT

Each skill should be taught in a logical progression from a simple to a more complex form. A suggested progression for dribbling, receiving, and flicking is outlined below.

Dribbling

1. Grip—stationary dribble
2. Dribble on the move with changes of speed
3. Use changes of direction: forward, backward, left, and right

Receiving

1. Stationary receiving balls from straight on, left, right, and behind
2. Receiving balls from each direction while on the move
3. Controlling of balls hit at various speeds

Drive

1. Stationary—straight, left, right, reverse stick
2. Dribble and drive in different directions
3. Drive for accuracy

Flick

1. Stationary—varying heights
2. Flicking on the move
3. Flicking for accuracy

DRILLS TO DEVELOP PROPER TECHNIQUE

There are many drills and variations of drills that can be used to teach each of the techniques. A few are presented here with the intent of providing a logical progression with an emphasis in technique needed to avoid injury.

Dribbling: Emphasize looking up

1. The ball is placed on a line. A player push dribbles the ball forward along the line while looking up.
2. The player dribbles the ball forward about three yards then stops the feet and the ball, looks up, then continues three more yards.
3. The player stands straddling a line with the ball on the line. Rotating the stick over the top of the ball from right to left and back again, the player alternately plays the ball with a face stick or reverse stick over the line.
4. The player dribbles forward, backward, left, or right on verbal command.
5. Same as 4, but visual command.

Receiving: Emphasize controlling the ball on the stick

1. Pairs. Partners stand about 10 yards apart. One player pushes the ball to the other who attempts to receive it under control. Once the ball is controlled it is passed back to the first player.
2. Same as 1, but the ball is pushed to the left or right of the player, forcing movement to receive.
3. Same as 1, but with a controlled hit.
4. Same as 2, but with a controlled hit.
5. Pairs: receiving on the move from the right and left. Player A passes the ball forward for B to run onto. B receives the ball, dribbles beyond, and stops. B then passes forward for A to receive. Change direction to receive from the right.

Driving: Emphasize firm wrists and keeping stick head below shoulder height.

1. Pairs: practice proper technique while driving the ball back and forth.
2. Same as 1, but with drives to the left and right.
3. Threes: in a shuttle relay formation with one ball. Dribble and hit

the ball to the opposite person. Move to the end of the opposite line.
4. Same as 3, but with drives to left and right.
5. Pairs: players stand 10 yards apart and drive the ball to each other attempting to place it through two cones one yard apart (accuracy).

Flicking: Emphasize accuracy and control of the height of the ball.

1. Pairs: flick back and forth keeping the ball about six inches off the ground.
2. Same as 1, but use a variety of heights.
3. Threes: A and C are 20 yards apart with B in between. A flicks the ball past B to C. C receives and flicks back to A. Change the middle person.
4. Pairs: one player dribbles the ball forward and flicks it to the other.
5. Same as 4, but vary the speed and height of the ball.

PHYSICAL REQUIREMENTS OF THE ACTIVITY

As in any game that involves extensive running, proper conditioning is important in preventing catastrophic injury due primarily to loss of body control. Field hockey is similar to soccer in that it is a fall sport, and therefore, the athlete needs to train over the summer to be in top physical condition at the beginning of the season. The athlete should be given a summer conditioning program designed to provide a solid base of endurance. The athlete should be warned of the risks involved in returning to practice without proper conditioning and encouraged to train as much as possible over the summer. The coach should remember that not all athletes will train with intensity. Therefore, the fall conditioning program should be realistically based on the returning level of fitness of the players.

SPECIAL SAFETY CONSIDERATIONS

Rules of Play

The rules of hockey have generally changed to reflect safety concerns. The increased use of aerial balls in game play resulted in potentially hazardous situations, and the rules were modified to limit their use. The interpretations of the rules also changed. Balls lifted into groups of people were considered dangerous; therefore, the player responsible for lifting the ball was penalized. When a player improperly fielded a ball causing it to rebound in the air, the player was assessed the foul for not controlling the ball.

A rule that presently seems to be interpreted less stringently with respect to safety consciousness than in the past is that of "high sticks." The rule states that a player may not raise the stick above shoulder height on either the backswing or the follow-through. The current interpretation is to let the play continue unless the player is using high sticks in an intimidating or dangerous manner. The use of the stick is considered dangerous when another player is in close proximity. The result has been an increase in the number of athletes raising their sticks dangerously high, which creates greater risks of players being struck in the head. While this may not be a severe problem for more advanced players, it is imperative that beginners be taught proper technique, and that a strong emphasis be placed on keeping the head of the stick below shoulder height.

Safety Equipment

As in soccer, the rules state that a player shall not wear anything that is dangerous to another player. Again, the major concern is that footwear not have any dangerously protruding spikes or nails. No special safety equipment is required, although many athletes choose to wear mouth guards. This is a recommended practice even though failure to wear a protective device would not result in catastrophic injury.

Of particular concern should be the protection of the goalkeeper, who is in a vulnerable position since lofted shots and rebounds off sticks are common in the goal area. It is essential that the goalkeeper be trained in the proper techniques of fielding an aerial ball. It is also critical that the goalkeeper be provided with adequate protective equipment. It is becoming a common practice for the goalie to wear a face mask in addition to the traditional pads and gloves. See Chapter 10 on ice hockey for further equipment safety concepts.

A final safety concern relates to the care and repair of sticks. Sticks should be periodically checked for splinters and cracks. Under no circumstances should a player be allowed to play with a broken stick. It is possible that a player could be seriously injured if struck by the head of a stick that has become detached from the shaft.

Playing Field

Prior to practice and play, the field should be checked for holes, debris, water, and other hazards to unsuspecting players. Uneven footing creates the potential for falling and uncontrolled movements that might result in catastrophic injury.

9

Football

STEVE MORTON
Washington State University
Pullman, Washington

Many statistics are kept in the sport of football. This benefits fans, players, and coaches. One area of statistics kept is on the injuries that occur during the season. They are never as glamorous as the game statistics, but nonetheless, they are real.

In 1982, data available revealed there were 24 catastrophic injuries and seven deaths involved in football at these levels: youth, inter-scholastic, and intercollegiate (Mueller and Blyth 1983). Torg et al. (1985) reported the cervical quadriplegia data for the years 1971 through 1984. A marked decrease of cases was noted: 34 cases in 1976 and five cases in 1984 causing permanent quadriplegia. There was a total of nine cra-niocerebral deaths. Although this is a very small percentage of partici-pants, many other people are affected, such as family, friends, and coaches. These catastrophic injuries, their causes, some preventative measures, and safety hints will be discussed in this chapter (Table 9-1).

POSSIBLE CATASTROPHIC INJURIES

Since blocking and tackling are basically the same technique, they will be looked at simultaneously. The most common injuries occurring during blocking and tackling involve the head and neck. One of these, the concussion, can lead to brain damage or death. A cervical injury to vertebrae one through seven can cause paraplegia, quadriplegia or even death. Blocking and tackling with the head down (neck in flexed posi-tion) and hitting an opponent's thigh or knee or hitting the ground can cause one or both of these injuries. Also, blocking and tackling with the head hyperextended while hitting an opponent's thigh, knee, or the ground can result in catastrophic head and neck injury.

Table 9-1. Possible Catastrophic Injuries in Football

Activity Skill Technique	Possible Injury(s)	Cause(s)	Prevention: Proper Instruction	Safety Hints
Blocking, tackling	Cervical injury (vertebrae 1-7), Paraplegia, Quadriplegia, Death	Blocking or tackling with head down, neck in flexed position, Hitting knee or thigh, Blocking or tackling with head in hyperextension, Hit square with head in numbers of opponent	Head and eyes up (hit with shoulders), Keep hips under center of gravity (prevents spearing)	Proper fitting and approved equipment, Drills to teach proper techniques, Neck exercises to strengthen neck muscles, Strict adherence to rules
	Concussion, Brain damage, Death	Hitting or being hit by opponent's head, knee, thigh or ground	Same as above	Same as above
Being speared	Broken ribs, Punctured lungs, Kidney damage, Spleen damage	Being speared by opponent in mid-section or back	Rules, Officials	Use of "flack jacket" or similar protection
Karate chop (clothes-lining)	Cervical injury	Striking head or neck with extended forearm	Rules, Officials	Does not apply

WARNINGS

With this in mind, every athlete should be warned of the possible dangers involved in performing the techniques improperly. In addition, since collisions among players occur frequently and are inherent in the sport of football, the athlete and the parents or guardian should also be notified both in writing and verbally of the potential dangers in participation in the game of football. This notice should state that the coaches are aware of potential danger and will use proper methods to teach the techniques of blocking and tackling. There is, however, no guarantee that a catastrophic injury, including paraplegia or quadriplegia, will not occur.

INSTRUCTORS' RESPONSIBILITY: TEACHING

Basic instruction should include keeping the head and eyes up during blocking and tackling and making all initial contact with the shoulders. It should also be stressed that on contact, the best position for the hips is under the center of gravity. This will aid in body contact and help prevent spearing.

There are many excellent blocking and tackling drills used to practice the proper techniques in blocking and tackling. The biggest considerations in the selection of the drills are the skill level and the physical condition of the athlete.

It is very important, regardless of the skill level of the athlete, that the neck be strengthened as much as possible. This can be accomplished by the use of many exercises such as the "wrestler's bridge" or an isometric/isotonic combination neck workout. No matter which method or methods are used to strengthen the neck, the full range of motion must be conditioned.

A logical approach to the sequence of blocking and tackling drills should be planned. At no time should a full-speed drill be used before a proper warm-up routine. Also, one should never go straight to a line blocking or tackling drill without first going through a half-speed simulation of the technique. This gives the athlete a chance to "get a feel" of the techniques desired. This will also enable the coach to correct the athlete and respond to any questions concerning the drill or the techniques.

The rules concerning blocking and tackling have been made to protect the blocker, tackler, and the opponent. Although these rules will vary greatly from Little League or Pee Wee football on up to the professional rank, at *NO* time should a coach bend these rules. Strict adherence to all rules will not only help protect the players, but also help protect the coach if a catastrophic injury should occur. Therefore, a coach must teach sound and safe techniques and make sure there is a clear understanding of limitations via rules with respect to techniques. Unsafe coaching techniques and inadequate comprehension and application of the rules constitute grounds for a case in a court of law.

EQUIPMENT AND FACILITY RESPONSIBILITIES

There is a military saying that goes like this: "A soldier's best friend is his rifle." Change a couple of words and you can adapt this saying to fit football. It could read: "A football player's best friend is his equipment." The equipment directly involved with blocking and tackling are the helmet and shoulder pads. Both of these items may be satisfactory when they are manufactured, but they will wear and deteriorate. The proper inspection of both is the duty of the coach or equipment manager. Regardless of who has the responsibility of inspection, it should be done regularly. Any equipment found defective can be replaced or rebuilt and sent on for subsequent safety certification. All helmets must have the NOCSAE label on them. It is also important that the athletes be instructed on how to inspect their own equipment for wear.

In addition to proper selection and maintenance, equipment must fit correctly and be used properly. There are many instruction manuals that can be obtained through equipment manufacturers, which illustrate the fitting of all football equipment. The coach should be able to fit and advise the athlete in the correct usage of each piece of equipment. The equipment manager and trainer (if applicable to the situation) should also know how to fit equipment. Both coach and athlete must be made aware of any special fittings (i.e. use of air in an air helmet and the importance of maintaining the precise level of inflation to achieve maximum protection).

The next step to aid in the prevention against catastrophic injury is to inspect the practice and playing fields. The field should be free of holes, debris, and other hazards. All goal posts should be padded. Before beginning a drill, inspect the adjacent area. Any walls that could be struck by players running or falling out of bounds should be cushioned. If doubts arise about what is considered a safety hazard, consult other coaches, trainers, or sports facilities experts.

RULES FOR SAFE PLAY

Make sure the terminology used in a playbook, or in the description of a drill, is worded technically. The following is an example: use "shoulder block" instead of "spear block," or "perfect form tackling" rather than "head-hunter drill." Always be conscious of what is either written or spoken. Remember, these terms can be used in a court of law.

There are two other areas of concern on the topic of catastrophic injury in football. The first is being "speared" by an opponent. The second is a karate chop, or clotheslining-type tackle. Although the player being "speared" or "clotheslined" has no control over the opponent's action, catastrophic injury may result to one, or both, players.

In the case of "spearing," the ensuing injury to the "spearer" could be of the head and neck variety described earlier in this chapter. The player being "speared" in the midsection or back can receive either broken ribs (which can result in a punctured lung), kidney damage, or spleen damage.

Prevention of these injuries is in the hands of the coaches. No coach should ever condone the act of "spearing." Warn the athlete of the potential danger to both parties involved. As a coach, one should know the rules surrounding all the techniques that are being coached.

A rib protector or "flack jacket" are the only pieces of equipment available to aid in the prevention of injuries involving the midsection. The most important protection is the coach insisting on strict adherence to the rules, and the officials' enforcement of those rules. If there is a problem of spearing within a league or division, it should be brought to the attention of the Officials Association. When the officials enforce the rules as they are written, the game will be safer and more fun.

The "clothesline" tackle is not only against the rules, it is very dangerous to the athlete being tackled. Again, the cervical area of the spine is the site of greatest potential danger. This technique should *never* be taught, encouraged, or tolerated.

The only preventative measures available are the rules governing the use of this technique. If a problem arises within your league or conference, the matter should be taken to the Officials Association. Here, the problem can be addressed, and the matter solved by either more awareness on the officials' part, or by bringing more emphasis of the problem to the coaches.

Following is an example of a staff statement and player rules used by the football staff at Washington State University. It may be advisable to do something similar and make it available to athletes and their parents or guardians. Perhaps the parental/guardian permission form would be an excellent location for this type of message.

W.S.U. COACHING STAFF STATEMENT

The Washington State University coaching staff condemns any act by a player to deliberately injure an opponent or teammate during a game or practice. The techniques taught to you by the coaching staff are designed to minimize the risk of injury to you and to your opponent.

The protective equipment you wear is the finest available and should not be abused by you. It is for your protection and should not be used in any manner as a weapon against an opponent or teammate. Of particular importance is the football helmet. When used properly, it protects you. When used improperly, it can become a dangerous weapon to you and to your opponent. The helmet should never be used to deliberately strike or hurt an opponent.

The following are some specific rules relating to the conduct and safety of our game. It is important for you to know these rules and adhere strictly to them. Unethical conduct and acts of unsportsmanship, whether within the rules or not, will not be tolerated by the coaching staff. Play the game hard, with enthusiasm and with intensity; but play it within the spirit and letter of these rules. Win with character!!

Rule: No person shall *strike* an opponent with his fist, or deliver a blow with extended forearm, elbow, or kick or knee an opponent during the game or between periods.

Rule: No player shall *meet* an opponent with the knee or strike an opponent's head, neck or face with an extended forearm, elbow, palm or the heel, back or side of the open hand during the game or between periods.

Rule: There shall be no piling on, falling on, or throwing the body on an opponent after the ball becomes dead.

Penalty: 15 yards and possible disqualification.

Use of Headgear

Rule: No player shall deliberately use his helmet to butt or ram an opponent.

Rule: There shall be no spearing.

Rule: No player shall intentionally strike a runner with the crown or top of his helmet.

Penalty: 15 yards and possible disqualification.

PRIDE—POISE—TEAM.
"CLASS IS PRIDE"

10

Ice Hockey

COSMO CASTALDI
University of Connecticut
Farmington, Connecticut

The severity and frequency of ice hockey injuries are not precisely known because organized hockey, like most sports today, is not involved in monitoring and recording the injuries of its participants.

Nationally, the Consumer Product Safety Comminssion (CPSC) has established the **National Electronic Injury Surveillance System** (NEISS), which collects data on all injuries including competitive and recreational sports. The NEISS program is a representative sample of about 5,000 hospital emergency rooms in the continental United States (Damron 1981).

The NEISS system also includes reference to protective equipment. Its most recent report, "Overview of Sports Related Injuries to Persons 5-14 Years of Age" (CPSC 1981), includes eye and spinal injuries as defined in this book. It does not include deaths of which there were two for the period 1973 through 1981.

Through the collaborative effort of colleges and high schools in the United States, the **National Athletic Injury Reporting System** (NAIRS) was established at Pennsylvania State University in 1974 and has collected data on some 30 different varsity sports from more than 200 colleges and high schools. NAIRS defines athletic injuries as follows:

1. **Minor Case:** Any reportable injury/illness (other than dental injuries) which did not keep an athlete from participation longer than one week.
2. **Significant Case:** Any injury/illness that kept an athlete from participation longer than one week plus dental injuries regardless of time loss.

3. **Major Case:** Any significant injury/illness that kept an athlete from participation longer than three weeks.
4. **Severe Case:** Any significant injury/illness causing societally serious disability (e.g., death, quadriplegia, amputation).

The definition of *severe case* seems to correspond with the designation of catastrophic injury as described in this work.

From the seven seasons between 1975 and 1982, an average of only seven institutions per year participated in the collection of data for ice hockey at the college level, a rather small sample from the total of more than 150 existing college hockey teams. Table 10-1 shows a rate of head, neck, and spine injuries which varies from 4.28 percent in 1977-78 to 12.21 percent in 1980-81. But Table 10-2 indicates that during the same period, there were no catastrophic injuries. Of interest, the injuries per exposure seemed to be declining slightly, most likely due to the introduction of a mandatory face guard rule with the 1978-79 season.

CATASTROPHIC EYE INJURIES

Although NAIRS data seem to suggest that catastrophic injuries in ice hockey are rare and that the game is becoming safer to play, recent reports from Canada are not so encouraging. Pashby reported that catastrophic eye injuries continue to occur on a fairly large scale (1981). Statistics compiled by the Canadian Ophthalmological Society for the period 1974-1982 (Table 10-3) showed that the number of catastrophic eye injuries in ice hockey were almost four times as high as in all other Canadian sports combined.

The value of a certified face mask in preventing eye injuries is beyond doubt (Table 10-4).

Whereas in 1972-73, the numbers of blinded eyes varies only slightly between age groups, by 1981-82, there was a dramatic drop in the under 16 year category, but a 40 percent increase in those over 16 years of age (Canadian Standards Association 1982). There are two reasons for this remarkable change: 1) the introduction of a mandatory face mask rule for players under 16, and 2) a phenomenal increase in the popularity of "Old Timers" hockey leagues whose participants are not required to wear a face mask.

During the period under study, *no* serious eye injuries occurred to players wearing the Canadian Standards Association (CSA) certified face masks. Examples of two masks, one which passes both the CSA 262.2 (Canadian Standards Association n.d. 1) and the American Society of Testing and Materials (ASTM F517.81) face guard standards (American Society of Testing Materials n.d. 1), and one which does not, are seen in Figures 10-1 and 10-2.

Table 10-1. NAIRS Ice Hockey Injury Rates

Body Parts Season:	Head, Neck, Spine	Head, Non-neurologic	Face	Shoulder, Arm	Forearm, Hand	Torso	Hip, Leg	Knee	Foot, Ankle	# of Teams Reporting	# of Games
1975-76	5.20%	2.31%	37.20%	9.50%	6.93%	5.20%	12.14%	15.03%	6.64%	9	301
1976-77	5.93%	0.79%	33.99%	12.64%	6.32%	11.07%	9.88%	11.46%	7.90%	6	190
1977-78	4.28%	1.56%	29.18%	9.73%	12.06%	7.78%	17.12%	14.00%	3.50%	10	286
1978-79	12.08%	0	19.76%	12.08%	7.69%	4.39%	12.08%	27.47%	4.40%	5	171
1979-80	6.06%	0	24.24%	12.12%	5.05%	11.11%	17.17%	10.10%	14.14%	5	148
1980-81	12.21%	0	13.74%	24.42%	8.39%	9.16%	10.69%	9.92%	10.69%	6	131
1981-82	9.62%	0	11.23%	19.25%	17.25%	7.49%	12.30%	17.25%	5.89%	7	187

Table 10-2. NAIRS Ice Hockey Injury Rates
Injury Severity Index/1,000 Exposures

Season	Minor*	Significant	Major	Severe	Injuries per 1,000 Exposures
1975-76	9.02	2.36	0.64	0	32.29
1976-77	10.75	2.90	0.92	0	33.84
1977-78	7.05	2.42	0.80	0	26.55
1978-79	4.02	2.12	0.80	0	15.17
1979-80	4.27	1.79	0.64	0	19.09
1980-81	5.49	2.32	1.11	0	20.23
1981-82	5.78	2.11	0.96	0	24.02

*Definitions given in the text.

Table 10-3. Eye Injuries in Canadian Sports, 1974-1982

Sports	Eye Injuries	Blinded Eyes
Hockey	1,000	154
Racquet sports	348	12
Ball hockey	100	7
Baseball	89	13
Football	31	1
Golf	12	5
Skiing	8	5
Broomball	9	2
Snowmobiling	4	2
Volleyball	14	3

Table 10-4. Eye Injuries in Canadian Ice Hockey

Age	1972-73	1981-82
up to 10	40	2
11 - 15	54	9
16 - 20	56	30
21 +	30	75

HEAD INJURIES

Concussion

The inclusion of concussion, particularly of the mild type, as a catastrophic injury might be questioned. However, repeated incidents of mild concussion must be included because of the possibility of adverse effects on the brain at some future date. Concussion can easily occur in ice hockey as the result of a blow to the jaw from a body check, or from a stick. It can also result from a fall to ice, against the boards, or from a

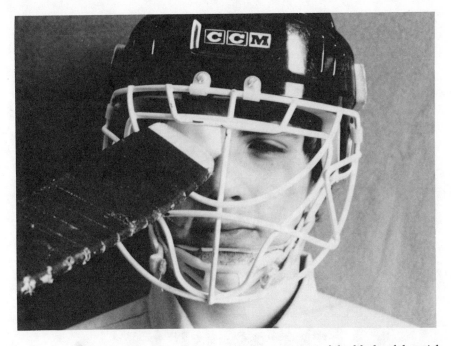

Figure 10-1 Hockey face mask which permits penetration of the blade of the stick in the eye area and also about the jaw. This mask does not meet the requirements of the CSA 262.2 or ASTM F517.81 standards.

collision with the goal or another player. Such impacts are of the high mass, low velocity type and are either preventable or greatly reduced in severity by the combined use of a certified hockey helmet (CSA 261.1) (Canadian Standards Association n.d. 2), and an internal mouth guard which meets ASTM standard F697-80 (American Society of Testing Materials n.d. 2). However, there have been isolated reports of concussions resulting from puck shots in players who were wearing certified helmets. Such an impact is of the low mass, high velocity type and has raised questions about the need for a more conservative standard to meet the ever increasing velocities at which modern ice hockey players are able to shoot the pucks.

Depressed Skull Fracture

This catastrophic injury was not so rare before the advent of the modern certified hockey helmet. In the National Hockey League, there was the famous case in the 1930s of "Ace" Bailey of the Toronto Maple Leafs who was heavily checked to the ice by Eddy Shore of the Boston Bruins. Bailey recovered from his injury, but Bob Masterton of the Min-

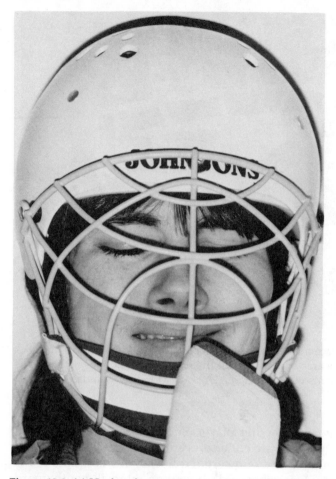

Figure 10-2 (a) Hockey face mask which does not permit penetration of the blade of the stick in the eye area. (b) Note that the blade of the stick is also prevented from penetrating the periphery of the mask. This mask meets the requirements of CSA 262.2 and ASTM F517-81.

nesota North Stars was not so fortunate. He died from a similar type of injury in 1967. Various types of certified hockey helmets are seen in (Figure 10-3).

Although all amateur and college teams require their players to wear helmets, the professional leagues do not, and about 10 percent of professional players choose not to wear them. In March, 1983, Ed Kea of the St. Louis Blues, who did not wear a helmet, sustained a depressed skull fracture in a Central Hockey League game and remained in a coma for two weeks after the accident. Four hours of surgery were required to

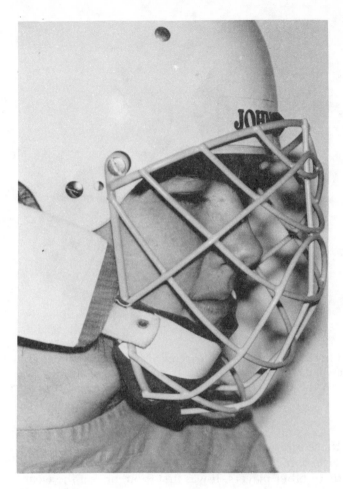

Figure 10-2b.

relieve pressure on his brain. To date, no depressed skull fracture injuries have been reported in players wearing hockey helmets certified as per the CSA hockey helmet standard 262.1-1975.

SPINAL CORD INJURIES

Until 1980, spinal cord injuries were very rare in ice hockey. Since then, however, there has been a rash of these catastrophic injuries in Canada, particularly in the Province of Ontario, where 12 significant cervical spine injuries have been reported. The players involved ranged in age from 16 to 20 years, and all wore helmets. Seven of the players were rendered either quadriplegic or paraplegic, while the other five suffered lesser trauma from which they have recovered (Bishop et al.

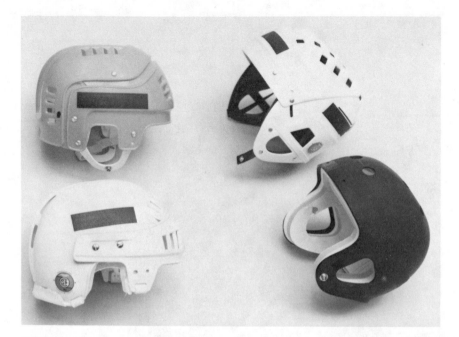

Figure 10-3 Certified hockey helmets. All four helmets are of different designs but each will pass CSA Standard 262.1. Note, however, that the two helmets on the right offer somewhat better protection in the ear area.

1983). A review of these injuries indicates that the permanent ones were of the "flexion-hyperflexion" type, and were the result of head-first collision with the boards or other players. It was first thought that the wearing of a helmet with a wire face guard might contribute to these cervical spine injuries. Three of the players wore helmets without a face guard. However, on the basis of skating studies and stimulated hockey checking forces applied to helmet-face guard combinations under laboratory conditions, Bishop et al. (1983) were unable to implicate the protective equipment as a significant contributing factor.

Other reasons suggested as contributing to these catastrophic spinal injuries are the increased size and speed of today's players and the presence of better protective equipment which gives the players feelings of invincibility and, therefore, greater willingness to take risks.

Other possibilities are failure to enlarge the size of the ice surface in accordance with the increased size and speed of today's players, the increase in rough play, and failure of officials to rigidly enforce the rules on rough play.

While the use of a certified helmet as per CSA Z262.1-M83 (Canadian Standards Association n.d. 2) cannot absolutely assure the prevention of concussion or catastrophic spine injuries, it is the best known method for reducing the possibility of such injuries.

SKATE CUT INJURIES

The severing of a nerve or major vessel, or the loss of an eye from a skate blade are all catastrophic injuries. Some of these injuries may be very difficult to prevent, but modern hockey skates include injury protective factors in the design of both the boot and the blade.

Injuries from the Front and Rear End of Skate Blades

The skate blade is inherently dangerous not only on the sharpened skating surface, but also at the front and rear ends. Prior to the modern plastic-metal blade combinations (Figure 10-4) hockey skate blades were all metal. The rear end of the metal blades caused many serious tear type injuries until organized ice hockey required a plastic protective guard to be attached to the rear end of the blade (Figure 10-4). Although a few players still wear the all-metal blade, almost all use the plastic-metal one.

These new blades appeared during the 1977-78 season and gained instant acceptance because of their lighter weight. However, the early models were very prone to breakage, and hockey skate manufacturers proposed that ASTM develop an ice hockey skate blade standard. One portion of the standard, ASTM 737-81, assures that the blade will stand up to the rigors of the game and not break as easily as did the first plastic-metal blades. The other aspect of the standard is concerned with safety and requires a one-quarter inch extension of plastic beyond the rear end of the blade. Although the ASTM standard for ice hockey skate blades has been in existence since 1980, many blades being used during the 1982-83 season did not pass the standard (Figure 10-4).

It is obvious that the rear end and possibly the front end of the all-metal blade can enter the eye and potentially cause blindness. The rear end design of the new plastic-metal blades appears less likely to cause such an injury, but depending on the design of the blade and the angle of impact, some might be more hazardous than others. The matter of compliance by organized hockey to existing standards for protective equipment can be considered a critical matter in the face of more legal suits from injured athletes (Adams 1982).

FALLS

Many of the injuries described thus far may result from falls to the ice or against the boards. Some falls are due to dull skates or deep cracks and/or cuts on the ice surface. Therefore, the importance of sharp skates and a smooth ice surface must be considered in the prevention of falls

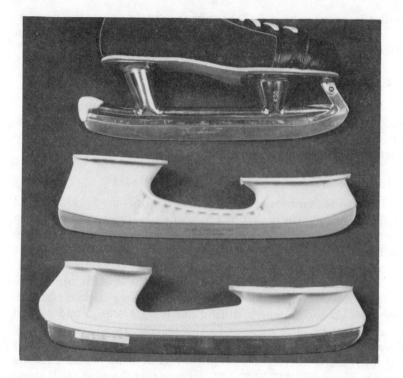

Figure 10-4. Hockey skate blades. The top blade is all metal and has a plastic protective tip (required by the playing rules) at the rear of the blade to prevent cut or tear injuries. The middle and bottom blades have metal runners and plastic holders. Note that the holder of the bottom blade extends beyond the runner at both ends. The bottom blade conforms with the ASTM F737-81 standard for skate blades, while the middle one does not.

which might lead to catastrophic injuries. Not only must players have their skates sharpened regularly, but the rink must not have exposed cement or metal in areas where players have to walk or stand on skates (corridors, benches, or penalty boxes), because of the possibility of ruining a sharp edge, thus contributing to a fall.

NECK INJURIES

Kim Crouch, a young Canadian goalkeeper, was fortunate to have survived a cut from a skate blade which penetrated his carotid artery. There was also the experience of a young goalkeeper in the Hartford Amateur Hockey League who was knocked unconscious when a rising puck shot hit his carotid sinus and rendered him unilaterally paralyzed within minutes. The timely intervention of an anesthesiologist, who just happened to be present, probably saved the player's life.

Although goalkeepers are the least injured of all ice hockey players, specialized protective equipment has been developed to prevent injuries in the neck area. The "Kim Crouch Collar" consists of a heavily padded protector which completely surrounds the neck and affords excellent protection against skate cuts. Like many baseball catchers, more and more goalkeepers are beginning to use rigid polycarbonate shields, which are attached to the bottom of their face masks and hang loosely in front of the neck.

RUPTURED ORGANS IN THE ABDOMINAL AREA

While the heart and lungs are natrually protected by the rib cage, the anatomical parts of the abdomen are more vulnerable. In particular, the liver and spleen are very susceptible to injury from the stick, the puck, a body check, or a puncture wound from a skate blade. Ruptured spleen injuries are not so rare in hockey, and if not diagnosed and treated properly, they can be catastrophic. In the past, hockey equipment afforded very little protection for abdominal injuries. Lately, however, the protective girdle and the extension of the shoulder pad to cover the abdominal area offers much better protection, and their use is highly recommended (Figure 10-5).

CARDIAC ARREST

While cardiac arrest is unlikely to occur in the young player, such is not the case for the older participant. There were incidents during the 1950 to 1960 period when older professional players suffered cardiac arrests during preseason training camps. With the modern emphasis on year-round conditioning and the insistence by highly competitive teams that their players report to training camp in superb condition, the possibility of cardiac arrest has been greatly reduced. But with the increasing interest in "Old Timers" hockey, the problem of cardiac arrest becomes a serious matter and underscores the importance of a preseason physical examination for such veteran participants.

BLOCKAGE OF AIRWAY

Blockage of the airway for more than 30 seconds will lead to anoxia, and if blockage is prolonged beyond four or five minutes, can cause severe brain damage and death. Such an injury can result from a skate cut or a severe blow to the neck. The possibility of airway blockage from swallowing a poorly fitted mouthguard also needs to be considered. In a review of 55 cases of sudden death from food asphyxiation in victims who choked on oversized pieces of meat, Haugen (1963) found the aver-

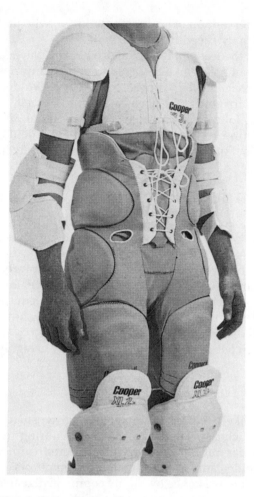

Figure 10-5a. The girdle which is designed to protect the hip area and much of the abdomen. Since 1981 when it first became available, there has been a significant decrease in hip and thigh contusion injuries.

age size of the impacted meat approached that of a package of cigarettes, which is much larger then many internal mouthguards. ASTM F697-80 Standard Practice for Care and Use of Mouthguards requires that the resilient plastic cover all the teeth of one jaw. Thus, the use of a cut-down loose mouthguard increases the possibility of asphyxiation. If a loose fitting stock mouthguard is used, the player should be informed about the potential of it being swallowed. Either the mouthguard should

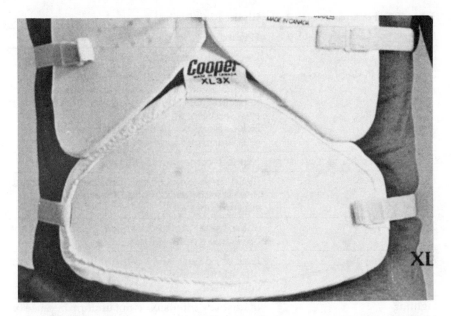

Figure 10-5b. Shoulder pad extension affords protection to the abdomen and is highly recommended for defensemen.

be replaced by one which fits well, or it must be attached to the player's face guard.

INJURIES DUE TO UNSAFE PLAYING FACILITIES

The potential of the playing facility contributing to a catastrophic injury in ice hockey cannot be ignored. In 1979, a young player was rendered unconscious and suffered severe brain damage when he was checked along the boards and an exposed portion of his head struck a metal upright from which some of the protective padding had broken away. Tom Webster, a top professional, had his career ended following a severe back injury. During a practice session, he collided with a goal post and unknowingly damaged a skate blade. When he rose from the ice and attempted to skate away quickly, the blade gave way and he fell a second time, resulting in the back injury. Whether such rare injuries can be attributed entirely to rink facilities may be debatable, but the need for safety standards for hockey rinks is an important consideration if the game is to become safer. Kemp (n.d.) has reviewed the rink facility regarding its potential for contributing to injuries and has alerted coaches about their responsibilities (Table 10-5).

Table 10-5. Hazards Associated with the Rink Facility

Item	Hazard
Ice Surface	Deep skate cuts and/or cracks
Players and Penalty Boxes	Gates which open out onto the ice surface; inadequate gate hinges and latches; large spaces between gates and ice surface and/or boards; exposed cement, or metal, or slippery floors; lack of plexiglass protection for penalty box area; improper location of boxes.
Dressing Rooms and Corridors	Exposed cement or metal, or slippery floors.
Enclosure	Ill-fitting sections of boards or plexiglass or outdoor screens, lack of padding around metal support posts.
Goal	Sharp metal protrusions, goal posts that do not break away upon impact.
Air Quality	Lack of exhaust fans or air conditioning to clear off carbon monoxide from ice resurfacing equipment.
Lighting	Inadequate intensity or not uniform because of poor design or burnt out bulbs.
First Aid	Lack of supplies, lack of easy access to first aid supplies and/or areas, inconvenient telephone for contacting ambulance, physician, or hospital.
Spectators	Throwing objects onto the ice surface.

RESPONSIBILITIES OF INSTRUCTIONAL STAFF AND ADMINISTRATION

No longer can educators, instructors, coaches, and even administrators limit their activities to organizing sports and improving players' individual and team skills. Recent court decisions make it abundantly clear that there is a responsibility which involves not only being knowledgeable about all aspects of the game, and particularly the hazards, but also to clearly inform the participants about the potential injury associated with those hazards (Adams 1982).

Responsibilities toward participants start long before the player takes to the ice. The following items are fundamental and should be considered sequentially:

1. Health of the players.
2. Condition of the playing facility.
3. Insurance coverage.
4. Protective equipment.

5. Off-ice preparation.
6. Warm-up procedures.
7. Specific skills training.
8. Team training for game conditions.
9. Cooling off procedures.
10. Knowledge of the playing rules.

Kemp (n.d.) has thoroughly reviewed the basic concepts of ice hockey, not specifically for the prevention of catastrophic injuries, but for all injuries, minor and major. What follows is a review of his recommendations.

Health of the Player

Coaches, parents, and the player must know what the player's physical condition is *before* any participation occurs. A physical examination by a physician must be obtained before the season starts to determine whether the player can withstand the strenuous nature of the sport. The instructor must be informed about any potential health hazards that might be aggravated by the planned instructional program. In the case of a minor, it is the parents' or guardian's responsibility to so inform the instructor.

All participants need not be perfect physical specimens, but it is the responsibility of the instructor to establish the appropriate training program and game participation within the limits of the player's health (Kemp n.d.) and even the player's size. It may be advisiable to have a 150-pound 12-year-old participant in the Bantam Division (13-14 years) rather than with his peers in the Pee Wee Division (11-12 years).

Insurance Coverage

While almost all participants will have some form of health insurance, compensation for accidents of a catastrophic nature is usually not included. Accident insurance over and above normal health insurance coverage is relatively inexpensive, and is highly recommended for coaches and game officials, as well as for the players.

Condition of the Playing Facility

Table 6-5 outlines most of the hazards associated with hockey rinks. While Kemp has alerted both coaches and players to study the rink facility prior to its use, he has not considered the responsibility of the rink management in reducing the hazards. The need for minimum standards for hockey rinks to reduce the possibility of injury to players seems obvious and is presently under consideration by the Ice Hockey Subcommittee of the American Society of Testing and Materials (ASTM n.d. 3).

Off-ice Preparation

Stretching exercises are important before any ice activity to slowly condition muscles and tendons prior to the more stressful anaerobic activity that follows. Players who are 15 years of age and older, have advanced skills, and will participate on highly competitive teams should have a *minimum* of two weeks daily graduated dry land training before the skating program begins.

Protective Equipment

For optimum protection against catastrophic injury, full protective equipment must be worn *at all times*, and every piece of equipment must fit properly. The helmet must fit snugly on the head, and the mouthguard must fit properly to remain firmly in place and not interfere with air exchange, as stock mouthguards are prone to do (Hayes 1977). In a preference test of *custom made, mouth-formed, or stock type* mouthguards, 87 percent of the users (high school football players) preferred the custom made type (Castaldi 1981).

All safety specification standards for protective equipment used in the game of ice hockey which originate in Committee F8 Sports Equipment and Facilities of the ASTM must include the following introductive statement:

> Ice hockey is a contact sport with intrinsic hazards. Protective equipment cannot eliminate all injuries, but will substantially reduce their severity and frequency. Participation in this sport by a player implies acceptance of some injury risk. The goal of protective equipment is to minimize the risk of injury.

Thus, it is clear that the recommendations made in Table 10-6 do not absolutely guarantee protection against catastrophic ice hockey injuries. Nor does the author endorse any particular product. Rather, the recommendations are considered to be the best available methods of protection today. Table 10-6 can serve as convenient check-list for instructional staff and participants.

Warm-up Procedures

A five-minute warm-up skating drill is mandatory before more intensive drills begin. Jean Belliveau, NHL Hall of Fame player, recommended the following warm-up drill as one which simulates game conditions and helps prevent groin pull injuries, which are notoriously slow to heal.

Players begin skating at a sustained slow speed with long strides and alternate leg, gentle stretching exercises while skating. This is continued for three laps around the circumference of the rink. Bursts of speed are then introduced from blue line to blue line with reduction to

Table 10-6. Catastrophic Ice Hockey Injuries and Recommended Protective Equipment

Injury	Protective Equipment and Designated Standard
Eye:	Faceguard as per ASTM F513-81 or CSA 262.2
Skull: Concussion, fracture	Helmet as per CSA 262.1 combined with internal mouth-guard as per ASTM F697-80.
Ruptures in abdominal area:	Shoulder pad extension to abdominal area.
Skate Blade Cuts: Achilles Tendon	Hockey boot incorporating Achilles tendon guard.
Neck	Throat collar, throat guard.
Face	Faceguard as per ASTM 513.81 or CSA 262.2.
Other body parts	Well fitted full protective equipment: faceguard, helmet, shoulder pads, elbow pads, pants, protective cup, shin guards, and gloves appropriate for the age/size of the player and caliber of competition. Skate blades to conform with ASTM F737-81.

slower speeds around the end zones. The procedure is then repeated in a counter clockwise direction. Table 10-7 offers some general guidelines for the instructional staff.

Specific Skills Training, Team Training, and Cooling Down Procedures

Every drill should simulate game conditions so that the participant learns to adjust quickly to the unexpected, and thus reduce the possibility of injury. Although recommended procedures will vary greatly between coaches, most coaches and instructors follow those listed in Table 10-7.

Role of Officials

Relative to other competitive sports, ice hockey can be considered a difficult game to officiate. Body contact is permitted by players moving at high speed in a playing facility which is not particularly large and which is bound by a rigid enclosure. In addition, hockey sticks, pucks, and skates can contribute to catastrophic injuries.

While organized hockey repeatedly cautions its referees about "letting the game get out of hand," it is well known that some officials are more lax than others in calling infractions. Furthermore, because the outcome of a crucial game may be decided by one team having to play shorthanded because of a penalty, it is easy to understand why officials might tend to ignore infractions, particularly during the last period of a championship game. The safety of players must be the prime considera-

Table 10-7. Practice Drills and Coaching Responsibilities to Prevent or Minimize Injuries

Drill	Responsibilities
All Drills	Full protective equipment, rink gates closed and latched, drinking water easily available, players fully recovered from previous injury, mandatory slow, warm-up skating drill before any other activity.
Skating	Properly fitted skates with sharp blades, slow warm-ups and adequate conditioning, padding on boards when teaching novice players to stop when skating toward the boards, periodic rests during drills, maximum of 30 skaters plus four goalies on ice at one time.
Shooting	No defective or illegal sticks, controlled shooting drills only, no shots higher than goal cross bar, keep shots low and soft to warm up goalie. Never allow two players to shoot simultaneously at the goalie.
Checking	Minimum body contact during practice sessions.
Scrimmage	Full protective equipment, controlled scrimmages, and only after thorough warm-up drills.
Cooling Down	Five minutes before the end of the scheduled ice time, all strenuous drills should be discontinued, after which players should skate slowly around the rink before retiring to the dressing room. This cooling down procedure will occur more effectively in the cooler environment of the rink than in the dressing room and is intended to help dissipate body heat and speed up a return to normal physiological conditions following the workout.

tion. In order to act responsibly in the prevention of catastrophic injuries, organized hockey (including the coaches) has the responsibility to:

1. Thoroughly inform officials about their responsibilities in calling infractions as they occur, regardless of the outcome of the game;
2. Weed out those officials who have a reputation for being lax in calling infractions, and
3. Support those officials who make unpopular decisions in situations where the referee's primary concern is player safety.

Recent lawsuits brought against organized hockey and its referees by players who have suffered catastrophic injuries make it abundantly clear that every effort must be taken to assure that the game of ice hockey is as safe as is possible for the participants without drastically altering its basic characteristics.

Knowledge of the Playing Rules

Knowledge of the rules is not only for game officials. Many rules pertain to injury protection, and coaches are obligated to familiarize themselves with the rules which govern their respective leagues, whether recreational, highly competitive amateur, scholastic, or professional.

SUMMARY

Ice hockey is considered to be the fastest team sport, and one in which catastrophic injuries can occur. While the introduction of modern protective equipment has helped, catastrophic injuries do occur. Reducing the number and severity of these catastrophic injuries is the responsibility of individuals who teach, coach, referee, or administer the game. Only through a sustained, committed effort on the part of all such individuals, in cooperation with health care professionals, scientists, designers, and standards setting organizations, will the game maintain respectability and continue to enjoy public support.

11

Rowing

GENE DOWERS
Washington State University
Pullman, Washington

The sport of rowing, or crew, is generally a very safe activity. The participants are separated and supported by their boats, and their body motion is basically linear in nature, eliminating major twisting and joint torsions. The most common rowing injuries are to muscles and connective tissue from overuse. These are best avoided through proper warm-up, stretching, and conditioning progressions. Catastrophic injuries are the result of the aquatic nature of the sport, the equipment, and the physical demands of the activity (Table 11-1).

POSSIBLE CATASTROPHIC INJURIES IN ROWING

1. Drowning
2. Gross injuries to muscle tissue, bones, and nerves (including the spinal cord) due to penetration of the bow stem of the boat (also called the shell) during collisions.
3. Injury or loss of the eye due to penetration of oars, rigging, and shell ends during the transportation of equipment.
4. Heat-related conditions including hypothermia and heatstroke.

Common Causes of the Injuries Above

1. Drowning most commonly occurs after a boat capsizes, or is swamped, or after a rower has been ejected from a boat. Ejection is usually the result of the rower losing control of the oar and failing to extract it from the water. When the blade doesn't come out of the water, the handle can strike the rower's body and the shell's momentum can cause the rower to be thrown over the side of the shell, or "catch a crab." Secondary drownings may also occur from the aspiration of either fresh or saltwater.

Table 11-1. Possible Catastrophic Injuries in Rowing

Activity	Possible Injury	Cause	Prevention
Immersion in very cold water	Hypothermia, Drowning	Capsizing, Swamping, "Catching a crab"	Swimming tests, Cold water survival instruction, Use of flotation devices, Use of safety launches, Technique training and attentiveness to rowing
Collision with other boats	Gross injury to bone, muscle, and nerve tissue, including the spinal cord	Insufficient caution in "blind boats," Inadequate bow ball	Establish and enforce rules for traffic patterns. Install effective bow balls on all shells. Accompany all "blind boats." Row with a coxswain, if possible
Rowing in high heat and humidity	Heat illness, including heat stroke	Fluid and electrolyte depletion, Inadequate acclimatization	Be aware of temperature and humidity. Allow fluid and electrolyte replacement. Allow rest and time to adapt to heat
Collisions with equipment during transportation or while stored	Damage or loss of the eye	Inadequate escorts and warnings while moving boats, Poor design of storage facilities	Escort both ends of all shells. Provide loud, clear, verbal warnings in crowds. Keep storage areas free of clutter. Pad all protruding surfaces

2. The bow stem of most rowing shells is extremely sharp and dangerous (Figure 11-1). Even when padded with most standard bow balls, damage can occur as the point of the shell will often penetrate through the bow ball (Figure 11-2). When two shells collide head-on or at or near right angles, the bow of one may penetrate the side of the other and will often strike the rower. This can often occur in shells without coxswains. These shells are referred to as "blind boats," since the oarsmen are seated facing the stern and cannot see where they are going without turning around.

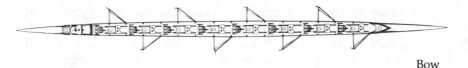

Bow

Figure 11-1. Bow stem of rowing shell.

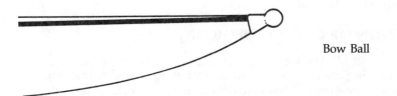

Bow Ball

Figure 11-2. Bow ball.

3. During practice or at rowing regattas, there are instances where oarsmen or spectators may be hit or run into by oars (Figure 11-3) and boat parts. The fact that shells are traditionally carried at head or shoulder height is a prime contributor to this problem. Collisions also occur inside boat houses where individuals may run into equipment on storage racks. Many shell houses are poorly lighted, and rowing equipment tends to be long, thin, and pointed. Any inattention in storage areas can lead to serious injury.

4. Hypothermia is the result of prolonged immersion in cold water, usually due to the same type of accident that causes drowning. This situation is often aggravated by lack of proper instruction in cold-water survival techniques and the absence of personal flotation devices. Heatstroke is totally avoidable and is usually the result of poor acclimatization and practice planning. Extended

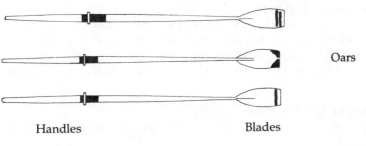

Oars

Handles   Blades

Figure 11-3. Rowing oars.

endurance rows and intense interval training on hot days with inadequate fluid and electrolyte replacement and rest may result in heat illness. Because most crews are composed of several rowers, coaches and trainers must be aware of the range of fitness and heat tolerance of the individuals in their care and insure that practice sessions do not overtax the least prepared. Humidity is always greater on a body of water, and practices must be planned accordingly.

PREVENTION OF CATASTROPHIC INJURY

1. **Prevention of Drowning**
   A. Swimming ability of each participant should be documented.
   B. All rowers should have instruction in safety techniques:
      - No rower or coxswain should ever leave their flotation or shell to swim for shore
      - A motor launch should stay within 100 yards of all shells when the air temperature is below 40 degrees F. or the water temperature is below 50 degrees F.
      - Shells without accompanying launches should keep within reach of shore in case it becomes necessary to swim to land (using the shell and oars for flotation on the way)
      - Shells rowing at night should be accompanied by a beacon-carrying launch
      - Weather forecasts and conditions, and, where applicable, tide schedules should be known by coaches and participants
      - Scullers and crews should report out and, in questionable weather, use a buddy system when not accompanied by a launch
      - Rescue procedures should be taught and practiced
   C. All coaches should be trained in lifesaving techniques and cardiopulmonary resuscitation (CPR).
   D. Wooden oars are Coast Guard-approved personal flotation devices. Plastic and aluminum oars may not have sufficient buoyancy to serve this purpose. All participants should be aware of their oars' ability to keep them afloat.
   E. Coxswains should be equipped with track shoes as footstretchers, and shoelaces should be replaced with quick-releasing Velcro closures to prevent oarsmen from being trapped under overturned shells (United States Rowing Association 1985).

2. **Prevention of Injuries from Collisions**
   A. Established traffic patterns for the body of water should be enforced.

B. "Blind Boats" should be accompanied by a launch whenever possible.

C. All shells should be equipped with non-collapsing, non-penetrable bow balls.

D. Oarsmen in "blind boats" should be instructed in steering and encouraged to take time to turn around and check the water ahead at regular intervals.

3. Prevention of Penetrating Injuries to the Eye

A. When carrying oars to and from the storage racks, the oarsmen should always keep the blades low and in plain sight. Oars should not be carried over the shoulder or with the blades to the rear.

B. Rowers should not carry more equipment than they can safely handle, i.e., no more than two oars at a time.

C. When a shell is being carried at head or shoulder height, individuals should be stationed at each end of the shell to "run interference" and ward off unsuspecting bystanders.

D. On-land traffic patterns should keep bystanders away from the top of docks and ramps and from the entrances of boat storage bays.

E. Coxswains and individuals monitoring the ends of shells being carried to and from the water should provide loud, clear, verbal warnings when entering or leaving boat bays and when entering crowds of spectators at regattas.

F. Equipment storage facilities should be designed to minimize traffic flow around equipment racks (also see Chapter 2).

G. Cluttered storage conditions that could lead to people standing up or turning around into protrusions on rowing gear should be eliminated.

H. All protruding surfaces should be marked and padded.

4. Prevention of Heat-Related Injuries

A. Instruction to prevent or reduce hypothermic reactions due to immersion in cold water should include (Collins 1976):
   - The head should be kept out of the water, i.e., DON'T DROWNPROOF
   - Unless land is within easy reach, holding still in the water is preferable to swimming or other vigorous activity
   - The Heat Escape Lessening Position (HELP) and Huddle procedures can cover areas of high heat loss and lead to increased survival time
   - The victim should get out of the water onto a log or upturned boat, if possible, and

- A life jacket is not really a life jacket unless it provides some measure of thermal protection.
B. Instruction to prevent or reduce problems due to overheating should include:
  - Know the warning signs and symptoms of heat illness,
  - Be aware of heat and humidity at the rowing site; a thermometer and an hygrometer are necessary,
  - Schedule practices to provide for fluid and electrolyte replacement and rest in conditions where prolonged exertion may be dangerous to the rowers, and allow time for acclimatization to hot environments.
C. First aid procedures for hypothermia and heat illness should be known (also see Chapter 3).
D. Coaches should know all emergency phone numbers and the locations of all telephones near practice and regatta sites.

CORRECT TECHNIQUE TO AVOID INJURY

Since the hazards outlined above do not result from the incorrect execution of the rowing motion, the teaching of proper technique has little to do with rowing safety. Some suggestions can be provided to reduce the chances of "catching a crab," such as inserting the blade into the water fully squared and avoiding feathering before extraction, but this will not eliminate the problem completely. More relevant is training rowers to be careful and fully aware of what is going on around them. Potential hazards must be indicated to these people at the outset and proper avoidance procedures suggested.

PHYSICAL REQUIREMENTS OF THE ACTIVITY

Rowing is primarily an endurance activity. It requires that the cardiovascular and respiratory systems be free from disease and defect and that these systems be trained progressively and in moderation. Physical examinations before participation begins will identify participants in poor health or with disqualifying conditions. Preliminary fitness testing will indicate the athlete's level of readiness for exertion.

Initial exertion should be of moderate intensity. Initial training bouts should be short and interspersed with rest periods. Duration of work can increase and rest decrease in a reasonable progression as indivduals adapt to the load. Intensity should not be increased until the individuals can continuously row fairly long periods of moderate work (30 minutes is suggested).

Because the body weight is supported by the shell, rowing is an activity that is well-suited for large individuals who have trouble moving their bulk against gravity. It should be noted, however, that rowing at high levels of output requires special attention to avoid heat illness. Beyond that, anyone with normal musculo-skeletal integrity and flexibility should have no physical problems with the sport.

SPECIAL SAFETY CONSIDERATIONS

Recommended Resource Plans: "MAN OVERBOARD!!"

Within the shell, coxswain in charge:
- "Weigh Enough!" (STOP).
- "Check it down!" or "Hold water!" (stop the shell/put on the "brakes").
- "Toss the jacket" (the coxswain tosses his/her life jacket to the victim).
- "Back it down!" (row back toward the victim).
- "Easy on the swimmer's side!" (row next to the victim).
- "Relax, hang onto the jacket, we're coming!" (establish verbal contact with the victim to calm and reassure them).
- Get the victim into the shell with the coxswain and transport to shore; do not let a hypothermia victim row; have the coxswain help them rewarm.

From the launch, coach in charge (American Red Cross 1974):
- Stop the practice with a pre-determined signal; all other shells should gather at the accident site.
- Toss a life jacket to the victim as soon as possible.
- Approach a victim from the down wind/down current side at minimum speed.
- Shut the launch's engine OFF.
- Establish contact with the victim; reach with a hand, pole, oar, or throwing line.
- DON'T GET IN THE WATER UNLESS ABSOLUTELY NO OTHER ALTERNATIVE EXISTS!!
- Move the victim to the stern of the launch to prevent capsizing.
- Get the victim out of the water and take him/her to shore. If assistance is needed in giving first aid for injury or hypothermia, take an oarsman (not the coxswain) from one of the shells. Get to shore as quickly as possible without leaving other crews unsupervised.

The rescue of multiple victims, as in a capsizing or swamping, assumes that the launch is large enough to hold them all safely and that there are enough life jackets for everyone in the water. The procedure is basically the same from there. Saving lives should always be more important than saving or recovering rowing equipment.

For the oarsman in the water:

- STAY WITH THE BOAT AND OARS; they will float even when full of water.
- DO NOT SWIM FOR SHORE; unless it is more dangerous to stay put, but then only go with flotation.
- HELP! (the Heat Escape Lessening Position) will minimize the body surface area which is exposed to the water. The knees are pulled up to the chest and the arms wrapped around the knees. Multiple victims should huddle together to minimize heat loss.
- Remain calm, stay still, keep the head out of the water, and signal distress.

12

Soccer

SANDRA MOORE
Kenyon College
Gambier, Ohio

Prevention of catastrophic injury begins with an awareness of the potential dangers inherent in the sport. When we think of serious injury in athletics, we think of the contact that occurs in football and ice hockey, or of the risks taken in gymnastics or diving. We often fail to realize, or see as significant, the potential for catastrophic injury that exists in other sports. Regardless of the probability of serious injury, coaches are responsible for understanding the risks involved in their sports, and for communicating the dangers to the athletes in their charge.

POSSIBLE CATASTROPHIC INJURIES IN SOCCER

Catastrophic injuries in soccer (Table 12-1) could include:
1. Spinal injury caused by failure to brace the neck properly when contacting the ball with the head.
2. Brain damage caused by an improper contact point of the head with the ball, or occurring when two players attempting to play the ball at the same time bang their heads together.
3. Tripping, causing a fall to the head or neck.

PREVENTION OF CATASTROPHIC INJURY

All participants should be warned that:
1. Lack of endurance training can lead to fatigue, indirectly causing injuries.
2. Flexibility and strength are important in preventing injury. Neck strength is crucial to safe performance in heading.
3. Extended periods of physical activity, particularly in warm

Table 12-1. Possible Catastrophic Injuries in Soccer

Skill	Injury	Cause	Proper Instruction	Safety Hints
Heading	Broken neck, Paraplegia, Quadriplegia, Death	Failure to brace neck on contact with ball	Tighten neck, tuck chin, and punch forehead at ball. Extend body back at waist and use neck muscles to direct ball	Drills: Toss ball to self first. Progress to partner tossing slow balls
	Loss of consciousness, Concussion, Brain damage, Death	Miscalculation of point of ball contact with head	Keep eyes on ball until it meets forehead. Keep eyes open throughout performance of skill. The midpoint of the ball should contact the forehead at the hairline. Always strike the ball, don't let it hit you	Rules: Don't push off an opponent for purpose of heading. Never charge an opponent who is in the air heading
Heading in game play	Loss of consciousness, Concussion, Brain damage, Death	Crashing of heads together in an attempt to play aerial ball	Body control. Awareness of others around. Close supervision of dangerous situations	Charging is legal but can be violent. Ball must be within playing distance. Player must have at least one foot on the ground. Hands and arms must not be employed to elbow or push. Point of contact is shoulder to shoulder
Heat	(covered in Chapter 3)			

weather, result in loss of body fluids that must be replaced, or heat exhaustion may occur. Athletes should be allowed frequent water breaks.

4. A blow to the head caused by a collision of two players, or incorrect ball contact during heading, can cause serious injury including brain damage.

5. Failure to tighten the neck muscles (brace the neck) while heading the ball can cause neck injuries which might result in paralysis.

6. Dangerous play can lead to serious injury.

CORRECT TECHNIQUE OF HEADING

Catastrophic injuries in soccer are rare, but the possibility exists that incorrect technique in heading could produce serious injury. Any part of the head may legally be used to contact the ball, but beginners should be taught to use the forehead. Anatomically, the forehead is the strongest part of the skull. Using the forehead also allows the eyes to follow the ball through contact. The flight of the ball is not always predictable, and the ball must be "led" to the forehead to ensure the proper point of contact.

In addition to the use of the forehead as the proper point of ball contact, the use of the neck muscles is a crucial factor in preventing serious injury. The speed of the ball coming at a player's head can forcibly snap the head back if the neck is not properly braced on contact. Players should be instructed to tighten to neck muscles and tuck the chin until the ball has been contacted. The head should be in line with the neck and trunk at the point of contact. This concept should be reinforced each time a new form of heading is introduced.

Heading the ball stationary or moving with feet on the ground at point of impact

In heading correctly, the player takes a stride position with the legs slightly flexed and the body inclined forward from the hips. The arms are held loosely forward for balance in preparation for contact with the ball. During the preparation, the body is moved backward from the hips. Prior to contact, the trunk swings forward with a powerful motion of the hips. The eyes remain fixed on the ball as it is "punched" by the forehead. At contact the legs straighten and a step forward is taken. There should be no movement in the head/neck joint.

Heading from a standing jump off two feet.

Start with the legs slightly apart. Flex both legs while swinging the arms backward and inclining the trunk forward. Take off by swinging the arms forward and upward while pushing from the ground as the legs straighten. The ball should be contacted at the height of the jump. The trunk is inclined slightly backwards and then moves quickly forward imparting power in a "punching" motion. The eyes remain fixed on the ball and balance should be maintained throughout. The landing should be on two feet with the knees and ankles "giving" to absorb the impact.

Heading a ball from a one-foot take-off after a short run

Using a five- to six-yard approach, the player gathers speed in a rhythmical run. Before the final liftoff, the trunk lowers and the body is pushed forward over the takeoff foot. The body weight rocks forward from the heel of the foot to the sole. On takeoff the support leg straightens. The other leg, which is flexed at the knee, swings upward with the arms helping to lift the body. At the top of the jump the trunk inclines backward. When the ball is at head height, the trunk moves forward giving power at impact. The landing is on both feet with the arms used to maintain balance.

PROGRESSION OF SKILL DEVELOPMENT

Heading should be taught in proper progression.
1. **Stationary**
   A. The players should practice bracing the neck and tucking the chin without the use of the ball.
   B. Again without the ball, players should practice the push of the knees forward and the movement of the trunk backwards. Add the straightening of the legs with the vigorous forward motion of the body.
   C. Practice the entire movement without the ball.
   D. Add a tossed ball attempting to head with a continuous motion. The eyes should watch the ball until it contacts the forehead. Gradually increase the speed of the incoming ball.
2. **Moving**
   A. Run, stop, and perform the skill from a stationary position as above.
   B. Attempt to head at a walk.
   C. Attempt to head while running.
3. **Jumping**
   A. Head ball from a jump off two feet.
   B. Head ball from a jump off one foot after a short run.

DRILLS TO DEVELOP PROPER TECHNIQUE

1. **Stationary**
   A. Toss ball to self about three feet over head—practice neck bracing and the proper point of contact.

B. Toss ball higher and add body motion.

C. Pairs: one partner throws the ball perpendicularly about three feet above head height. The other partner heads the descending ball back to the tosser. Change roles.

D. Same as C, but made more difficult by tossing the ball higher to increase the speed of the descending ball.

2. **Moving**

   A. Pairs: one partner tosses short high balls with a two-handed toss. The other partner runs into a position below the ball, stops, and heads the ball back. Change roles.

   B. Same as 1, but the ball is headed at a walk.

   C. Same as 1, but the ball is headed while running.

3. **Jump off two feet**

   A. Jump off two feet, practicing the body action without the ball.

   B. Toss the ball to yourself, then jump in the air and head the ball.

   C. Pairs: a tosser throws the ball with a two-handed toss in a steep arc from a distance of two to three yards. The partner jumps up and attempts to head the ball back to the tosser. Change places.

   D. Same as 3, but run, stop, and jump to head.

4. **Jump off one foot**

   A. After a short run of about three to four steps, the movement is performed without the ball.

   B. Pairs: a tosser stands about three to four yards away and throws the ball at a steep angle for the other partner to head back. Change roles.

PHYSICAL REQUIREMENTS OF THE ACTIVITY

Proper conditioning is a necessity for the safety of an athlete competing in soccer. Without proper endurance training, an athlete runs risk of catastrophic injury resulting from fatigue because of the stress placed on the cardiovascular system during extended periods of play. The risk is heightened by the fact that in most schools soccer is a fall sport, and many athletes are returning from a relaxing summer of inactivity.

Placing an athlete into a strenuous running activity without proper training can have catastrophic results. Because of fatigue, players may collide with other players, fall, and injure themselves and/or the other players. Therefore, the coach should meet with the athletes in the spring to emphasize the risks involved in returning to school without proper training, and to outline a general conditioning program for the athletes to follow during the summer. The running program should be of gradual intensity and designed to give the athlete a solid endurance base with which to begin the season.

It is imperative that the coach not assume that each athlete has diligently followed the conditioning program. Athletes have different motivations for training and in many cases do not train properly on their own. Lack of motivation, work schedules, or simply the fun and excitement of the summer can interfere with an athlete's best intentions to train. The coach should evaluate the level of fitness of the returning players and gear the preseason conditioning toward the establishment of the necessary level of cardiovascular endurance.

Conditioning for strength and flexibility is also important in preventing injury and should be included in the summer program. In terms of the prevention of catastrophic injury, particular attention should be placed on developing adequate neck strength to head safely. Some suggested exercises are as follows:

1. Pairs: Neck flexion. One player lies on her/his back and brings the chin to the chest while the partner applies a resisting downward pressure to the forehead. The pressure is great enough to cause strong muscle contraction and weak enough to allow movement to occur. Change positions.

2. Pairs: Neck extension. One player lies face down and raises the head as far back as possible while the partner applies a resisting downward pressure to the back of the head. The pressure is great enough to cause strong muscle contraction and weak enough to allow movement to occur. Change positions.

3. Pairs: Partners stand facing each other in a forward stride position. One grasps the other's neck with the right hand and attempts to bend the neck forward while the other resists the pull. The pressure must be regulated so that it is not too strong and is applied with the broad area of the hand. Repeat using the left hand. Change positions.

4. Pairs: One player stands with the legs spread, hands on hips, and trunk flexed forward. The partner stands opposite and leans with one or both hands on the back of the other's head. The first player attempts to raise the trunk, keeping the head in line with the trunk. Change positions.

5. Pairs: One player stands in a forward stride position while a partner stands in a similar stride position at the side. The partner grasps the neck of the first player with one hand and attempts to prevent the player from bending the neck in the opposite direction. Move to the opposite side and repeat. Change positions.

SPECIAL SAFETY CONSIDERATIONS

Rules of Play

To reduce the risk of serious injury, dangerous play should not be tolerated. The rules are designed to discourage rough play and limit body contact. Of particular concern is rough play that results when two players attempt to play an aerial ball at the same time (charging).

Charging an opponent is legal unless it is performed in a violent or dangerous manner. A fair charge is contact made with the near shoulder. In order to be legal, both players must be in an upright position and within playing distance of the ball. Also, both players must have their arms close to their bodies and must have at least one foot on the ground. The charge may not be violent nor made from behind an opponent.

In a game situation, the officials determine what constitutes rough play. They decide whether the charge is fair or illegal, and they have the responsibility of ensuring the safety of the players. In practice, the coach must be the enforcer. For the safety of all players, improper conduct or dangerous play in practice should be disciplined and then penalized as it would be in a game situation.

Safety Equipment

The rules state that a player shall not wear anything that is dangerous to another player. Footwear is a major consideration. Molded studs that are an integral part of the sole of the shoe should be made of rubber, plastic, polyurethane, or other soft material. The studs should be no smaller than ⅜ inch in diameter and should not protrude more than ¾ inch. Studs that are replaceable should be made of similar material and should be solid. The studs should be round and not less than ½ inch in diameter. No metal should be exposed on the sole of the shoe.

There isn't a rule that restricts the wearing of eyeglasses, but this practice can be dangerous. Players must be cautioned that the potential exists for the loss of vision. A player can be taught to turn the head on contact with the ball when heading, but this is not recommended as it encourages improper technique. The player should be urged to consider contact lenses or eyeglass protection. (See American Society for Testing of Materials [ASTM] standard recommended for racquetball.)

A final consideration is the danger inherent in the use of metal goalposts. The rules do not provide for the anchoring or padding of the goals for protection. Participants should be made aware of the risks involved in crashing headlong into solid metal goalposts. Horseplay should be prohibited, and the athletes should be properly supervised in practice.

13

Softball

TERRY COBLENTZ
Glendale College
Glendale, California

Softball is a game played on a field with two teams of nine active participants. The offensive team, or the team at bat, is attempting to score runs by hitting a pitched ball with great force, running around three bases and returning to the initial point, home base. The defensive team, or the team that is out in the field, is trying to prevent the offensive team from scoring runs by fielding the batted ball, often moving at high velocity, and throwing it, at high velocity, toward another player at one of the bases to which the offensive player is running. During these activities, there is some possibility of catastrophic injury (Table 13-1). Statistics indicate few catastrophic injuries in softball compared to some other sports. Even so, athletes and coaches participating in the game should take precautions.

POSSIBLE CATASTROPHIC INJURIES

Catastrophic injuries related to softball are similar to baseball, and include:

1. Loss of vision, paralysis, or death as a result of being struck in the head by a pitched, batted, or thrown ball, or by metal cleats.
2. Paralysis, death, or other permanent impairment of physical functions resulting from being struck by a bat, or colliding with another player or some part of the structure housing the playing field. Such impacts can result in injury to the head, neck, back, or specific organs. More persons have died from being struck in the chest than in the head in these sports. In particular, protection of the chest and vital organs is important to batters.

Table 13-1. Possible Catastrophic Injuries in Softball

Activity	Possible Injury	Cause	Prevention
Batting	Head or brain injury, Loss of sight, Organ damage	Being struck by the ball	Batting helmet, Alertness, Knowledge of moving away from a pitch
Baserunning	Head, neck, or back injury	Hit by a thrown ball, Collision with defensive player	Knowledge and application of rules and strategy, Alertness
Sliding	Head, neck, back, or organ injury	Collision with base or defensive player	Correct technique and appropriate use of skills
Fielding	Head, neck, organ, or eye injury	Collision with another player or obstacle, Being struck by the ball	Teamwork, "Calling" for the ball, Alertness, Appropriate positioning
Pitching	Head or eye injury	Being struck by a batted ball	Correct pitching technique and development of fielding skills

PREVENTION OF CATASTROPHIC INJURIES

Warning of Dangers and Dangerous Behavior

The following warnings should be clearly and specifically communicated to all players:

1. Lack of knowledge concerning the correct performance of the skills and of the game increases the possibility of injury.
2. Protective equipment is designed to reduce the risk of injuries to players. Not using it, or misusing it, takes away its effectiveness.
3. Protective equipment as well as other equipment that is broken or of inferior quality should not be used.
4. Lack of knowledge, misunderstanding, or improper use of the rules and strategies of the game increase the chance of injury.
5. Ineffective teamwork, such as not "calling" for a fly ball, puts players in a position of possible injury.
6. Throwing the bat after hitting a pitched ball puts others in a position of possible injury.
7. Being inattentive during a game results in increased chance of injury to the inattentive player as well as others.
8. Every playing field has potentially dangerous areas. Not know-

ing of possible "dangerous areas" and how to respond to them contributes to the possibility of injury during play.

CORRECT TECHNIQUE TO AVOID INJURY

General Fielding and Positioning Strategy

The cause of most injuries that occur in softball result from improper education of the players. There are many opportunities for an injury to occur during every aspect of play, and players from opposing teams increase the chances of injury-producing situations. Naturally, the base areas have great potential in this regard. Any time a play is made at a base, the fielder has to be sure that the baserunner has a clear path to the base.

At first base, for instance, the baseplayer should position himself or herself between the base and the thrower in order to catch the ball without interfering with the runner. The baseplayer's foot should be placed on the edge of the base as he/she catches the ball. Putting the foot in the middle of the base, or having the foot on the base when waiting for the ball, increases the potential for tripping the baserunner or contributing to a collision and resulting injury.

Second base is an area of high potential for injury, particularly during double play executions. The second base player should be instructed on how to receive the ball from a fielder and throw to first base without interfering with the runner. Also, players who must play second base position during double plays should have explicit instructions concerning avoidance of the runner's feet or body as the runner comes into the base.

Another area of high collision potential is home plate. The catcher is in a vulnerable position when a runner is attempting to score a run and a ball is being thrown to the catcher from a fielding position where the catcher cannot see both the ball and the runner. In these instances, the catcher must be positioned in front of home plate. If the ball is going to arrive before the runner, the catcher will move to a position over the baseline to tag the runner. The catcher should be instructed on the proper techniques for this situation to avoid a head-on collision while successfully tagging the runner or the base.

Batting

All players should be instructed in correct batting technique to avoid throwing the bat. In addition, the coach should provide for the use of gloves and wrapping or coatings of the bat to insure an adequate coefficient of friction during use of the bat.

Baserunning

Although fielding and positioning for baseplaying are very important, improper baserunning can also produce collisions or falls which result in catastrophic injury. Players should be knowledgeable of rules pertaining to the positioning rights of defensive players as well as the techniques of baseplay so that they "know where the baseplayer should be." In addition, they should be instructed in the correct techniques of baserunning.

Sliding is a part of baserunning and should be taught and practiced by all players. The potential for injury can be greatly reduced by the development of correct technique. (A discussion of types of sliding and drills for their practice is included in the baseball chapter.)

As with positioning and fielding strategies, an attitude of "making the play at any cost of self or another player," even if the rules can be "interpreted" to make it legal, should not be adopted. Having the spikes up, trying to roll into another player, or creating a head-on collision is inappropriate.

Pitching

The pitcher is in a particularly vulnerable position since that position is close to the batter, and the individual is completing the delivery movement toward home plate. Alertness and preparation for fielding a batted ball at the completion of the delivery should be included in instruction and practiced by all players.

Teamwork and Communication

Communication is important in reducing the possibility of injury as well as producing effective play. "Calling for the ball" is a simple skill, but can save players from life-threatening injury or death. This skill should be emphasized in the beginning stages of an athlete's career and reinforced as skill level increases. Players should be taught their territorial boundaries. For example, the infielder will always yield to the outfielder on a hit between them. It is, however, the responsibility of both players to communicate with each other, especially in situations in which both players might be able to make the play. If neither of the players "call for the ball" and both attempt to catch it, there may be a collision that could be catastrophic.

Being Attentive to Others and the Unexpected

Inattentiveness or "not thinking" are significant contributors to injury during play. Players must be prepared for the unexpected, or they are likely to respond in an inappropriate manner or fail to respond, increasing the chances of injury to themselves or to others.

Batting is a situation in which alertness is vital. Pitched balls approaching the body, especially the head and torso, should be avoided if possible. In such situations, batters should be taught to lower and turn the head away from the ball and use the arms to cover the torso. Ruptured spleens, stoppage of breathing from chest impacts, and kidney ruptures have been reported during baseball and softball play. Protective padding for the torso is being manufactured. It should be evaluated by teachers and coaches. Pitched balls that strike the torso or head may result in organ or cranial damage. If there is the slightest suspicion of organ or cranial damage, the coach should remove the player from the game or practice and secure medical attention.

Players should be coached to be alert also when on the bench, coaching, or not directly involved in the play. A broken or thrown bat, a "wildly" thrown ball, or a fast-moving player can create potential threats to safety. If all players are alerted to these situations usually no injury will occur. There are no drills, however, which can prepare players to anticipate all situations. They simply must be taught, and constantly reminded, to be alert and attentive to the circumstances of the game.

Drills

Drills used to teach the necessary offensive and defensive skills have to be very specific for the many situations that will arise at the various positions on the field. The age and skill level of the participants also should be taken into consideration. For example, a junior high school student without an extensive softball background will have to be taken step-by-step through a drill explaining the strategies included with the instruction. Since situations will change when there are runners on base or the ball and strike count of the batter changes, the drills must be "situational specific." An example of a situational drill is as follows:

> There is a runner on first base with one "out." The ball is hit to the first baseplayer, who is situated well in front of first base. Since a defensive player should never throw the ball across a basepath that has a runner involved, the shortstop moves to a position to the inside of the base to receive the throw. The shortstop then throws the ball to first base and completes the double play.

This drill keeps the defensive players out of the base paths of the offensive players, lessening the possibility of collisions and players being struck by the ball. Drills for a variety of situations should be practiced. Safety, as well as effective play, should be emphasized during instruction.

Progression of Skills

The pace of progression through skills should be determined by the coach's evaluation of the participant's skills and ability to learn new skills. Basic skills should be mastered before additional or more complex skills are included in instruction. There is no advantage in progressing any faster, since incomplete skills contribute to injury-producing situations.

PHYSICAL REQUIREMENTS OF THE ACTIVITY

The physical requirements of softball are not rigorous. A softball game usually lasts no longer than two hours. During that time only the pitcher and catcher are actively participating the majority of the time. The bases are 60 feet apart, and the longest run an offensive player will have to contend with is 240 feet interrupted by three 90-degree turns. The defensive team does not have a great amount of running to do during a play. The infielders cover a small territory, and an outfielder will never have more than about 80 feet of territory to cover. Nevertheless, the players should be conditioned so that short, intense movements can be executed without fatigue. Fatigue may cause loss of balance and control of movements, putting a player in a situation predisposing to injury. In addition, drills to enhance attentiveness should be a part of the conditioning regimen. Coaches should be alert to symptoms of heat stress, clouded vision, and waning of attentiveness on the part of players. Those players with such symptoms should be prohibited from further participation during that session.

SPECIAL SAFETY CONDITIONS

Rules of Play

The rules of play are written to prevent hazardous play. The baserunner's path is designed to prevent the runner from leaving the basepath to disrupt defensive players. Defensive players cannot block the baserunner's progress to a base, and the pitcher is not allowed to pitch "at a batter." Other rules, such as the Infield Fly Rule, were established to keep play competitive and safe. The Infield Fly Rule discourages an aggressive baserunner from running into the fielding player in an attempt to "break up the play." An understanding of the rules and their intent by both the coaches and the players contributes to safe play. Park and league personnel should establish their own ground rules to increase safety when deemed necessary.

Officials interpret and enforce the rules, further reducing the chance of injury to players. Coaches, however, should not place all the responsibility for monitoring safe play on the umpires. Coaches have responsibilities as well.

Safety Equipment

A minimal amount of safety equipment is required for softball. The catcher requires the most protective equipment; a mask with helmet and a body protector are the primary pieces. The helmet protects the catcher from serious head injury, whereas the mask is designed to prevent injury to the face. The body protector reduces the seriousness of blows to the chest or abdominal area. In fast-pitch-rules the batter is required to wear a batting helmet. The helmet reduces the force of any blow to the head as a result of a pitched ball.

It is the coach's responsibility to make certain that all safety equipment fits, and that it is of appropriate quality and undamaged. The batting helmet should cover the temples throughout any movement of the head. The catcher's mask must have openings small enough to prevent the ball from making contact with the face. During fast-pitch-rules, the throat and crown of the head should be protected as well. The body protector should fit so that it covers those areas most vulnerable to injury.

All equipment should be evaluated in terms of the most recent standards and specifications available. Evidence exists that masks that do not meet safety standards for prevention of ball penetration have been sold. The coach, before purchasing masks, should check their performance records. Unsafe masks, and other equipment deemed to be defective, should be returned to the company, and the ASTM F.8 Committee should be notified (1916 Race Street, Philadelphia). For further information concerning safety equipment read Chapters 2, 6, and 8.

Instructor Supervision

Whenever a team takes the field, it is the primary responsibility of the instructor to be certain that the athletes have had adequate training. The instructor should be aware of any unsafe or unique conditions related to the playing area and advise the players with respect to appropriate actions. Balls, bats, and other equipment should be inspected for safety and assurance of legality. In addition, the coach should dictate what takes place during the game, stay within the intent of the rules, and not manipulate the rules of the game so that unsafe circumstances result.

14

Team Handball

HASHEM KILANI
University of Jordan, Amman

LAURICE DEE
University of Illinois at Urbana-Champaign
Urbana-Champaign, Illinois

Team handball was originally played by track and field athletes in Europe as part of their conditioning program. Over the past 60 years, team handball, as a sport, has gained rapidly in popularity and is now being played in 75 nations by more than 3 million players affiliated with the International Handball Federation. The first international meet was held in September 1925, with Austria defeating Germany.

The transition of team handball from a conditioning program to a competitive sport over the years has proved to be both beneficial and detrimental to those who play. Athletes benefit from taking part in a sport that emphasizes overall body conditioning during exercise and competition. Additionally, they benefit from engaging in teamwork and learning highly refined fundamental skills from the highest levels of international competition.

One unfortunate aspect of team handball is the possibility of catastrophic injuries (Table 14-1). Such an occurrence might be due to the physical roughness of the sport at the national and international levels. For example, at least two deaths from head injuries in international team handball competition were reported in 1976.

Since team handball is a contact sport, coaches, teachers, and participants should be aware of the potential for roughness to those who play or practice the game. Catastrophic injuries are more likely to occur in those who do not follow the rules of safe team handball play

Coaches, teachers, and participants should take preventive measures to reduce the number of injuries in team handball. They also should

Table 14-1. Possible Catastrophic Injuries in Team Handball

Activity	Possible Injury	Cause	Prevention
A player's attempt to score a goal	Face, head, neck, or back injuries, Brain injury, Concussion; Paralysis, Loss of olfactory sense, sight, and hearing, Coma, Death	Improperly defended by opponent. Collision with other players. Improper landing to the floor after a lay-up (shot) to score a goal	Knowledge of moving away from an opponent. Quick decision making as to whether to score or pass the ball to a teammate (the decision depends on whether an attempted scorer is surrounded by opponents or the path to the goal is blocked by opponents). Correct technique and appropriate use of landing skills
Defending an opponent (i.e., prevent an opponent from scoring)	Face, head, back, or neck injury, Brain damage, Possible concussion, Paralysis, Coma, Death	Player collision, Improper fall to the floor, Improper defending technique obstruction	Correct technique and appropriate use of defending and landing skills
Blocking an opponent from scoring by the goal keeper	Same as above	Inappropriate positioning, Lack of alertness, Player collision, Improper defending technique, Being struck by the ball	Appropriate positioning. Alertness. Correct technique and appropriate use of defending, catching, and blocking skills

assist in the design and evaluation of playing surfaces and facilities that would be safer and benefical to players.

POSSIBLE CATASTROPHIC INJURIES

1. An attempted scorer may experience loss of sight; face, head, and/or neck injuries; brain damage; or possible concussion, when improperly·defended by an opponent.
2. An attempted scorer may experience catastrophic injuries to the neck, head, face and/or back; brain damage; possible concussion; paraplegia; quadriplegia; coma; or death when diving to the floor during a layup to score a goal and/or a collision with other players.

3. A defender may experience the same injuries mentioned in 1 and 2 when a collision occurs.
4. A goalkeeper may experience the same kind of injuries mentioned in 1 and 2 when ball contact and/or player or object collision occur.
5. If fluids are not administered during pratice or competition in hot humid weather (especially if team handball is played outdoors), and rest periods have not been scheduled, there is a possibility of death or illness as a result of heat stroke or heat exhaustion.

CHARACTERISTICS OF TEAM HANDBALL AS A SPORT

In the United States, people tend to confuse team handball with "handball," a game that is played in a closed court (a small enclosed room with four walls and a ceiling enclosing the room). The introduction of team handball as a sport can be confusing, as the sport is not as readily recognized in the United States as it is in Europe and the Middle East.

Team handball is played on a court similar to a basketball court. Each team has seven players (six players and a goalkeeper) who play both offense and defense. The basic objective is to throw the ball into the two by three-meter goal of the opponent and to defend one's own goal against attacks by the other team.

Team handball is quite easy to learn since the basic skills of running, jumping, catching and throwing are employed by the participants. The game is usually played at a quick pace by the participants of each team when the play is alternated from offense to defense (i.e., from one goal area to the other). The participants normally display quick bursts of energy in their movements by sprinting on the court, changing directions while sprinting, diving to the ground, and/or rolling on the ground to grasp the ball and/or throw the ball to a teammate or the goalkeeper. Such skills require anaerobic energy, which is the combustion of muscle glycogen without the presence of oxygen to provide energy for muscle contraction. These skills are utilized with the ball, a leather one weighing 425 grams and measuring 60 centimeters in diameter, held by one hand or two. Handling, passing, and shooting of the ball are also part of the team handball technique.

In countries where the weather is decent most of the year, team handball is usually played outside. Otherwise, this sport is played indoors.

Whether or not team handball is played indoors or outdoors, the playing surface is one of the criteria for the physical safety of the participants. The playing surface should be smooth, flat, and free of potholes.

The participants usually wear shorts (or sweat pants) and T-shirts for maximum comfort while playing team handball. Many participants wear protective knee and elbow pads. No special pair of shoes is required; the participants wear shoes that are comfortable for them (e.g., tennis shoes, running shoes, racquetball shoes, or basketball shoes) and produce adequate traction with respect to the playing surface. There soon will be team handball shoes especially designed for optimal performance and safety.

Simple rules are followed while team handball is played. They are as follows: players may dribble the ball, although the game is not as dribble-oriented as basketball; players are allowed three steps before and after a dribble, but while stationary, they may hold the ball for three seconds; body contact is allowed by the defense to stop the offense from scoring (however, the use of legs or arms to push, hold, trip, or hit is a violation, and excessive roughness results in two-minute penalties, as in hockey); internationally the game is played in two 30-minute halves with a 10-minute intermission (there are no timeouts); and the goalkeeper may defend the goal by using any part of his/her body.

CAUSES OF ROUGH PLAY IN TEAM HANDBALL

Team handball is considered a rough sport at the national and international levels, and roughness displayed by the participants has always been the nature of the sport. Physical violence has been exhibited by the players during practice and competition. Since body contact is allowed by the defensive team to prevent the offensive team from scoring, the development and onset of catastrophic injuries may be possible. Such injuries can occur as a result of physical forces that are exerted by players in an abusive manner.

Physical forces exerted by the participants involve body contact, and the most frequent body contact and vigorous play occur at the goal area line and the free throw line on the playing court. The reason for more frequent body contact at those two areas is due to the members of defense players trying to block the offense team during an attempt to score points by throwing the ball into the goal.

Blocking, however, is not the only cause of possible rough play or physical violence occurring on the court during practice or a game. Several other factors may be cited as causes of rough play by the participants on the court. They are listed as follows:
1. Insufficient physical fitness and lack of technical preparation of players may contribute to the frequency of injuries on the court through violence. Such players will experience difficult in mastering and controlling their actions, responding to quick stimuli from the playing environment, and executing proper skills during practice or competition. Additionally, the participants' desire to win may result in physical roughness (via body contact and collision with other participants) to compensate for their lack of proper physical fitness. As a result, roughness on the court may contribute to the development of cata-

strophic injuries. Another possibility is fatigue on the part of the participants. Participants may injure themselves or others through lack of physical coordination that has been precipitated by muscular and mental fatigue.

2. Lack of sportsmanship on the part of the participants may contribute to violence on the court. Such a lack of sportsmanship may include acts of degradation by participants on one another, especially during competition. In other words, they may go out to "get one another" by pushing, kicking, and shoving with intent to harm.

3. Lack of proper leadership and guidance on the part of the coaches, managers, teachers, and team organizers may contribute to the participants' lack of knowledge and understanding of proper conduct while competing on the court. A good example would be the loss of physical and mental control on the part of the player during competition when he/she becomes discouraged as a result of poor performance. Lack of control may cause players to take frustrations out on others through physical violence. The guidance and leadership of a coach is of paramount importance to control violence. A coach should stress that the game of team handball should not be conducted like war and no team includes a person who is an enemy. The coach should go further to point out that teams include only "rivals" whose aims are to display their superior playing abilities and physical conditions. A coach should serve as a role model. The behavior of players on the court is influenced mainly by how they have been treated by the coach. For example, an extremely agressive and revengeful attitude exhibited by the coach may influence the players to seek violence and revenge during practice and competition. A coach who is more of a moderator may aid the maintainance of proper conduct by players during competition.

4. Differences in culture and the personal background of coaches, players, and team organizers may contribute to the development of improper conduct during competition. Physical contact and violence on the part of players may be stressed and promoted more in some countries than in others, and the attitude of coaches and players toward the notion of "fair play" varies. People from some countries may consider the game of team handball as a "fight" by players who are involved in competition. For example, illegal use of legs and arms to push, shove, kick, and hold the opponents have been developed by the defense team to stop the opponents from scoring.

5. Inconsistent officiating and handling of team handball competition by the officials may contribute to the unsportsmanlike conduct on the part of the players who take part in the competition. When the game is not properly officiated, the game and the players' conduct may get out-of-hand, because rules regarding body contact have not been fol-

lowed. Referees who do not have complete control of the game seem to lack the sense of how team handball should be played. Therefore, the safety of the sport is undermined.

THE DEVELOPMENT AND ONSET OF INJURIES FROM PLAYING TEAM HANDBALL

The onset and development of team handball injuries may be due to intrinsic forces that have been exerted by the body, extrinsic forces that have been exerted on the body via body contact or collision with an implement, lack of mental and physical preparedness for competition, and lack of physical conditioning. There is a lack of research relating to the identification of the single factor that causes the most catastrophic injuries.

Blocking an opponent or the ball and jumping and landing after throwing the ball are the activities of handball that may lead to the most number of catastrophic injuries. Catastrophic injuries such as head, neck, spinal, and eye injuries; concussion; brain damage; paraplegia; quadriplegia; coma; and death may occur as a result of the following: initial landing occurs on the back, neck, shoulder, or head: players landing on top on one another during a fall; colliding of an attempted scorer and defender (e.g., one's elbow may accidentally hit another player directly in the eyes, nose, or ears causing possible loss of sight, olfactory sense, or hearing); and colliding of players or players and an object, such as the goal or ball.

CORRECT TECHNIQUES TO AVOID INJURY

Technique in team handball is the ability of a player to form intelligent rational movements which are shown in concrete motor actions during a game situation whether with a ball or without it. Tactics can be defined as the mental and physical preparation through systematic study and application of specific patterns of play for maximum efficiency (i.e., positive results). It is imperative here to master the technique (skills) before attempting to follow particular tactics. Therefore, a proper method should be provided for the individual as well as for the team to reduce the possibility of a catastrophic injury which may occur due to poor technique and poor tactics.

Injuries to a Potential Scorer

A potential scorer may experience loss of sight; face, head, and/or neck injuries; brain damage; or concussion when improperly defended by an opponent. In other words, the scorer may collide with an opponent or receive a blow to the eye, face, head, or neck from an opponent.

The following drills can be used to train shooters to avoid being hit by opponents and to reduce the frequency of body collision with opponents. Drills usually involve most of the elementary movements, and they are as follows: simple running and jumping; specific movements such as short dash; drawing opponent out of position; break-in; outrunning an opponent; screening; faking; falling; rolling; diving; and cushioning the fall with the palms of hands.

Locating Opponents Drill

A shooter should check where most of the opponents are as soon as the ball is received. If there are no opponents close and the path to the goal is clear, the shooter attempts to score. Otherwise, the shooter passes the ball to another teammate. This drill may be organized with three or more defensive players, one shooter, and one passer. The defense is free to move until the shooter receives the ball from the passer. All defense remain stable when the ball is passed and until the shooter decides what to do.

Cushioning Drill

Before a player attempts to score by way of diving into the goal area to shoot, he/she should check to be sure that nobody is in front of him/her. After releasing the ball, the shooter falls forward into a push-up position with the arms bending at the elbows to absorb the weight. This drill is designed to execute a diving attempt at the goal. The shot and dive are practiced without opponents and preferably on mats. After releasing the ball (simulation without ball should be practiced with unskilled players), the shooter falls forward into a push-up position with the arms bending at the elbows to absorb weight.

After the technique is learned, the drill is modified. A stationary opponent stands in front of the shooter. The shooter must shoot and dive to one side and forward to avoid the opponent.

Once again, more and more freedom is given to the defense as the shooter becomes more proficient. Although this should be practiced, care should be taken to observe the performance. Any sign of fatigue or difficulty in diving properly are indications to terminate the drill.

Throwing Drill

Throwing the ball is one of the fundamental skills of the game of team handball. The player must direct the ball accurately from one point to another. There are two objectives in throwing the ball: passing to a teammate and shooting for a goal. Shooting for a goal using a one-handed throw from above the head is the most common type of throw.

Maximum speed occurs as a result of using full body force during the follow-through phase of throwing. A whiplike action of the throwing arm is created by a player if full body forces are being used in sequence during the throw, and diving and rolling toward the floor are common after the release of the ball. A player, however, should avoid shooting directly at the goal keeper. Balls should be directed to the low and high corners of the goal area and rebounding shots off the floor during practice.

Gymnastic Tumbling Exercise

In order to perfect the shooting technique without an occurrence of a potential catastrophic injury, the shooter must learn how to cushion body contact with the floor. This skill is developed through gymnastic tumbling exercises.

The shooter should practice falling forward and landing on the hands with arms flexed at the elbows until confidence and proficiences are learned. This exercise should be practiced half of the time without throwing the ball (i.e., no ball in the hands) and the other half with the skill of throwing.

However, there are other ways of falling and absorbing weight, and the exercises to reduce injuries are as follows: after the ball is released, the body falls forward with the throwing arm and shoulder continuing the follow-through causing the body to roll sideways longitudinally upon contact with the ground. This rolling motion attenuates the impact force.

Coaching Points

Coaches should be sure that those who attempt to perform such risky tactics are experienced and courageous players.

Injuries to Both Defender and Goalkeeper

Both defender and goalkeeper may experience the same kind of injuries that an attempted scorer experiences when ball contact and/or player or object collision occurs.

The following drills can be used to train defenders to defend properly without colliding with other players, particularly an attempted scorer.

Ducking Drill

If an attempted scorer moves arms or legs in such a way that the defender may get hit in the face, head, or neck, the defender should duck the head and place the arms between the head and opponent. This defensive action should be practiced in groups of two. The offense player will raise the arm quickly in a simulated throw toward the defender's head. The defender immediately performs the "ducking action." This is repeated 10 or more times.

Sprinting Drill

Both the defender and goalkeeper should work on short and long sprints (forward, backward, and lateral sprints) so that they can keep up with the speed of the opposing team during an attempt to score. The goalkeeper practices with two opponents who pass the ball and move quickly, continually changing directions. The goalkeeper moves to the appropriate defense position.

Coaching Points
Coaches should be sure that players defending their opponents do not display any physical actions which are violent in nature. Otherwise, the number of injuries will increase as a result of such physical violence.

SPECIAL SAFETY CONSIDERATIONS

Rules of Play
For the purpose of preventing catastrophic injuries, rules regarding improper player conduct have been specifically identified with severe penalties for violations. Coaches and athletes need to know and understand the rules, and enforcement of the rules should be maintained at all times.

Safety Equipment
At the present time, the international team handball rules include no reference to protective equipment. Players usually wear no protective equipment. Coaches in the United States must use common sense in determining what equipment should be required.

Since head injuries of minor and major significance are common in team handball, protective helmets might be developed so that players' heads can be protected from hits, bumps and collisions with objects or other bodies. Protective helmets worn by team handball participants may resemble those boxers wear. Helmets should be well-ventilated, padded and should not impair vision or hearing. At this time, research has not been conducted on what type of helmets should be used.

The design of protective vest pads for the upper torsos of participants along with protective joint pads might be recommended by the coaches. The protective vest pads should be padded both inside and outside and cool enough for the participants to wear, especially when they sweat during competition. At this time, mouth protection and eye protection should be available and used by team handball players. Both are especially important to the goalkeeper.

Younger and less experienced players may be coached to shoot using jumping and stationary techniques without diving. Thus, protective equipment may not be necessary since players will remain upright.

As team handball gains in popularity, injury data should be reported and interpreted. Such procedures will provide a basis for modification of rules or introduction of protective equipment.

Awareness of Safety Measures in Team Handball by Coaches, Athletes, and Officials

In addition to knowing and understanding the rules, coaches and athletes must have knowledge of how violent or savage contact on the court may cause catastrophic injuries. In other words, they should be aware that swinging of arms and elbows, striking another person with the fist or elbow, excessive kicking and kneeing with the legs, running under a player who is airborne, and crouching or hipping in a manner which might cause an injury to an opponent should be prohibited.

With the knowledge of rules and the causes of catastrophic injuries in mind, the coaches and athletes will be aware of which bodily movements are the most violent and should be eliminated during team handball competition.

Coaches should be aware that fatigue on the part of players is a potential cause of catastrophic injuries, and players who display physical fatigue by not being able to control their movements on the court should be promptly removed from the game or workout. If the players are working out or playing a game outdoors, they should be given rest periods and plenty of fluids, especially when the weather is hot and the humidity level is high.

Coaches should check to be sure that the playing facility is a safe, well-lighted one and the equipment (i.e., goal nets and handballs) have been thoroughly inspected for possible defects. The floor should be inspected for cracks, wet spots, potholes and dirt, and any flaw that is detected on the floor should be immediately corrected and competition postponed.

Coaches and athletes are not the only ones who promote understanding of the nature of team handball as a rough sport and rules regarding body contact. Officials (specifically referees) should establish understanding of how team handball as a rough sport contributes to the development of catastrophic injuries on the part of the players.

Referees are responsible for the handling of competition. Games should be properly officiated by the adherence of existing team handball rules, and the conduct of the players should be kept under control at all times.

15

Volleyball

JIM COLEMAN
International Men's Volleyball Team
Walla Walla, Washington

MARLENE ADRIAN
University of Illinois at Urbana-Champaign
Urbana-Champaign, Illinois

Volleyball is one of the most popular participant sports in the world today. It is played at all levels of organization and by people in all walks of life. The game is best known by the bullet-like spikes and great diving saves made by the Olympic teams of Japan, China, the Soviet Union, and the United States, but it is more often enjoyed by friends and neighbors on a Sunday afternoon picnic.

Fortunately, volleyball is a relatively safe sport. The probability of a catastrophic injury occurring in volleyball is almost too small to calculate. Yet, serious injuries and death have occurred. Coaches, teachers, and participants need to be aware of the potential hazards of the game (Table 15-1).

POTENTIAL CATASTROPHIC INJURIES

Catastrophic injuries related to volleyball include:
1. Loss of eye caused by collision with volleyball net equipment or with other players.
2. Severe brain damage or spinal cord damage caused by collision with net support equipment, the floor, the walls, or other players.

WARNINGS OF DANGERS AND DANGEROUS BEHAVIOR

There are six types of situations that create serious hazards to volleyball players. These are:

Table 15-1. Possible Catastrophic Injuries in Volleyball

Activity	Possible Injury	Cause	Prevention
Collision with net equipment	Eye, Brain, Spinal column	Uncontrolled pursuit of the ball	Reminders to players of danger. Teaching of rules
Opposing players colliding at net	Brain damage, Death	Uncontrolled jump by blocker or spiker	Teach blocker to jump with control, no broad-jump. Spikers must never jump into net or over centerline
Player landing on floor	Cervical neck damage	Improper techniques for landing on the floor	Follow sound teaching progressions. Learn proper landing techniques. Use arms to cushion landing and prevent head from hitting floor
Player-to-player collisions	Eye, Brain, Spinal column	Unclear defensive strategies or uncontrolled player activity	Defensive areas of responsibility must be understood. Good judgment must be reinforced
Sustained vigorous action	Cardiorespiratory failure, Falling on head	Cardiovascular medical problem, Fatigue	Physical exam by physician. Proper cardiovascular conditioning. Stopping play when fatigued
Impact with net equipment	Eye, Brain	Unsafe equipment, Unsafe storage	Well-designed and safe equipment

1. Player collisions with the net and net support equipment.
2. Uncontrolled player-to-player collisions at the net between players on opposite teams.
3. Player collisions with the floor while attempting to play balls that are difficult to retrieve.
4. Uncontrolled player-to-player collisions between players on the same team.
5. Players who have exceeded their cardiovascular health and fitness levels.
6. Moisture on the floor.

COMMENTS ON THE CORRECT TECHNIQUES
TO PREVENT INJURIES

In the game of volleyball, a number of players move quickly within a confined space to pursue a ball which has been rapidly propelled by an opponent. The players need to be well trained, and the equipment needs to be well designed so that the possibility of injury is minimized.

1. Players should be both cautioned and trained to avoid collisions with nets, net support equipment, and official's stands. Spinal column injuries can occur as players run into guidewires supporting the net posts. Eye, brain, and spinal column injuries can occur as players collide with the net posts and official's stands.

2. The major possibility for serious injury occurs as opposing players are in competition at the net. Untrained blockers will lose body control and become entangled in the net, or they will step over the centerline under the net. At the same time, untrained spikers will fall or jump into the net and collide with the blockers. Players have not only been injured from collisions with opposing players, but also from the heavy net posts falling upon the entangled players. Brain damage and death have occurred in such instances.

3. Players are taught to dive and/or roll for balls that are difficult to retrieve. Two or more players colliding at high speed in an attempt to make these difficult plays are in danger of brain and spinal column injuries. These collisions may not be preventable since the athletes must be taught to play very aggressively, and yet the athletes must be taught to do this with control. Therefore, proper strategy must accompany the teaching of these aggressive defensive techniques so that collisions will not be with the head or neck. Each player must know his or her area of responsibility on each play so that player-to-player collisions can be avoided.

4. Players must be taught safe techniques for diving and rolling for the ball. There are a number of safe techniques. During the learning stages of volleyball, technique and player safety are most important and ball retrieval is secondary. Brain and cervical spinal injuries can occur when poor landing techniques are used.

5. Training for and playing volleyball can create stresses on the athlete's cardiovascular system. Volleyball players should be tested by a qualified physician and must be properly conditioned before being subjected to severe cardiovascular training bouts. Incidents of falling and general loss of body control are more probable in athletes with low levels of conditioning.

6. Coaches, players, and officials must check the surface of the floor for moisture as a result of perspiration "dripping from the players." Falling can result if the moisture is not wiped away.

COMMENTS ON TEACHING TECHNIQUES WITH EMPHASIS ON SAFETY

1. To the casual observer, it would seem obvious that an athlete would avoid collisions with net, the net posts, the other equipment which supports the posts and the official's stands. Unfortunately, untrained players must constantly be reminded that it is not only dangerous to hit the equipment, it is usually against the rules. It is common for spikers in warm-up to request sets that are very close to the net so they may smash the ball virtually downward. This often leads to the spiker either hitting the net or landing on the other side of the centerline. This practice becomes a habit which then becomes quite dangerous if carried out in competitive situations.

2. The situation in which opposing players interact at the net is a complicated situation involving blocking and spiking techniques, team strategy, and spatial awareness. Blockers must be trained to start very close to the net and to jump in a vertical line. Blockers should never use an approach to aid in jumping. Using an approach might cause that blocker to violate the net or the centerline and make contact with other players.

   Good spiking technique, on the other hand, encourages the spiker to broadjump (jump horizontally). In order to allow for the spiker's broadjump, the setter must set the ball sufficiently far away from the net so that the spiker may jump, hit the ball, and land without violation. If the set is too close to the net to allow for the broadjump, the spiker must be able to adjust the jump to avoid the broadjump and the violation. During learning situations in which either the spiker or blocker(s) is untrained, the players must be instructed to avoid jumping for the balls which are set very close to the net. This warning usually has to be repeated frequently.

3. Power volleyball requires a great deal of player-to-floor contact. Among the common techniques taught are the dive, the sprawl, the extension roll, the log (barrel) roll, and the cushioned roll. All of these techniques are good and are effective, although most players will learn only one or two of them. There are a few guidelines which are common to all of them. First, teaching sequences must be strictly followed. Second, the

player should begin in a low ready position and never raise from that position. The fall should never be more than 18 inches. Pictures of volleyball players flying through the air at unreasonable heights is not a practical image to give to an untrained player. Third, the fall should be cushioned by the arms, but the major force of landing should be borne by the large surfaces of the body. The part of the body absorbing the primary force of landing will vary depending upon the technique used. Proper landing techniques do not allow the head to be aimed at the floor. Cushioning with the arms should keep the head and chin away from floor contact. Players must demonstrate safe landing techniques in ideal situations without the ball before they are allowed to attempt to play the ball.

4. Once players have acquired diving and/or rolling skills, they must be taught to be both aggressive and controlled. Each player must know his or her defensive area of responsibility and must not impinge upon the defensive space of a teammate. Furthermore, the players must learn strategies when the ball is hit into a "seam" between areas of responsibility. For example, the line digger dives into the center of the court, whereas the deep digger dives parallel to the net, but deeper than the line digger.

CONSIDERATIONS FOR SAFE EQUIPMENT

The net standards and supporting equipment present the greatest hazard in the game of volleyball. Most net posts weigh between 20 and 100 pounds, are long and awkward to handle, have high centers of gravity, have protruding sharp objects, and have relatively large bases. All of these relatively necessary features of a net post present dangers for the participants.

Net posts are required to be positioned a minimum of three feet off the court. Participants should be instructed to keep away from them during play. Most commercially available net posts have form-fitted pads for player protection. It is wise to use these pads. Posts should be secured to the floor, or, preferably, inserted into the floor. Bolts and fittings need to be constantly monitored to be certain that they are in proper working order and can withstand the strain of play. In one instance, death occurred when a player fell into the net, after which the net post fell on the player's head. The floor-bolt had not been tightened sufficiently to maintain the net post in an upright position. All fittings should be checked before play is allowed.

Volleyball net posts are awkward to handle. All persons expected to move them should be properly trained. Free-standing net posts in storage areas may constitute a hazard. If the posts have a small base, they do not stand well when stored unsupported. These posts should be constrained in some manner. If the posts have a large base, they are awkward to move and present a hazard during play.

Unless net posts are inserted into the floor or fastened to the wall, they should be supported by guidewires. However, serious injuries have occurred when rapidly moving players have hit guidewires with their heads or necks. Therefore, the guidewires should be a safe distance off the court and should be cushioned and/or visibly marked.

Part III

Individual Sports

16

Bicycling

FRANK PETTIGREW
Kent State University
Kent, Ohio

The bicycling craze which began in the mid-1970s is almost certain to continue, as more people begin to discover the bike's advantages as a means of obtaining a level of fitness as well as a mode of inexpensive transportation. There have been more bicycles sold in the United States since 1970 than automobiles, with more than 100 million bicycles in use today. Manufacturers predicted that an excess of 10 million bicycles would be sold in 1985, making bicycling the most popular participant sport in the country.

Along with the increased number of bicycles and greater mileage per bike comes an increased number of injuries and deaths (Table 16-1). The National Safety Council reports that more than 1,000 people per year are killed in the United States as a result of collisions between bicycles and motor vehicles. In addition, 150 to 200 deaths per year can be attributed to non-motor vehicle collisions or falls. The National Safety Council estimates that of the one million bicycle injuries per year, approximately 70 percent require emergency room treatment. Ninety percent of all deaths are a result of some type of head injury.

POSSIBLE CATASTROPHIC INJURIES

Catastrophic injuries related to bicycling include:
1. Death—by having a collision with a motor vehicle, other bicyclists, or a a stationary object, which results in a fall due to loss of control.
2. Severe head and spinal cord injuries—obtained from the same causes as listed in 1, but resulting in temporary or permanent loss of physical and/or mental functioning due to trauma to the head region.

Table 16-1. Possible Catastrophic Injuries in Bicycling

Activity	Possible Injury	Cause	Prevention
Bike/car accident	Death, Severe head injury, Lacerations, Fractures, Abrasions, Contusions	Not paying attention when being overtaken by a motorist, or not having sufficient riding skills such as scanning, balance, and control	Pay attention to overtaking motorists. Develop riding skills that will enable the bicycle to stay under control and in a straight pathway at all times
		Bicyclist makes an unexpected turn or swerve	Be able to execute an emergency stop or a quick turn maneuver
		Bicyclist rides out into a controlled intersection	Obey traffic laws and signs, especially at intersections
			Wear a helmet
Bike/only accident	Death, Severe head injury, Lacerations, Fractures, Abrasions, Contusions	Loss of control leading to a fall or collision with a stationary object	Scan ahead for surface hazards and obstacles in the biking route
		Colliding with a stationary object with subsequent loss of control	Operate the bicycle at speeds which will ensure maximum control
		Colliding or having a near collision with a moving object	Be able to judge other road users' intentions, particularly other bicyclists

3. Lacerations, fractured bones, contusions, and/or abrasions—These injuries also are obtained from falls, and can vary from minor bruises and cuts to seriously debilitating medical problems for the bicyclist.
4. Dehydration—Due to the lack of drinking water or liquid while bicycling for long periods of time.

CLASSIFICATION OF ACCIDENTS

There are two distinct levels of bicycle accidents; 1) those that involve a bike and a car (bike/car) and 2) those that involve just the bicycle (bike/only). Bike/car accidents occur far less frequently than bike/only accidents, but they are responsible for almost all of the fatalities and a large percentage of the catastrophic injuries. Bike/only accidents refer to a bicycle hitting another bicycle, a pedestrian, or a fixed object. They also include a bicyclist losing control and falling due to deep gravel, ice, or oil on the road. Listed below are the three major types of accidents for each category.

Bike/car	*Bike/only*
1) Motorist overtakes bicyclist	1) Collision or near collision with moving object with subsequent loss of control
2) Bicyclist makes unexpected turn or swerve	
3) Bicyclist rides out into a controlled intersection	2) Loss of control leading to fall or collision with stationary object
	3) Collision with stationary object with subsequent loss of control

PREVENTION OF CATASTROPHIC INJURY

Catastrophic injuries in bicycling happen because someone does something wrong, and in more than 75 percent of the cases, it is the bicyclist who makes the mistake. In order to avoid such mistakes, a cyclist must be able to perform the following physical and mental skills. These skills should be mastered before bicyclists can be considered ready to ride anywhere in relative safety.

1. Allow motorists to overtake (come from behind) and develop the ability to judge the car's pathway without losing balance and control.
2. Execute an emergency stop and/or quick turn maneuver with control.
3. Obey traffic laws and signs, especially at roadway intersections.
4. Judge the intentions of other road users, particularly other bicyclists.
5. Operate at speeds which enable them to control their bicycles at all times.
6. Scan ahead for surface hazards, vehicles, animals, obstacles, or anything that might possibly affect one's travel.
7. Choose appropriate clothing for protection. This includes brightly colored clothes (fluorescent if riding at night) and a quality helmet.
8. Properly mount gear or pack so that it avoids the spokes or gears. Utilize tie downs or pannier bags to secure any items that are carried on the bicycle.

SPECIAL SAFETY CONSIDERATIONS

Bicycling can be a very dangerous physical activity . . . one careless act can prove fatal. Unlike most other physical activity, bicycling includes the unpredictable factor of traffic.

One of the most basic pieces of equipment for cyclists is a helmet. A safe, well-fitted helmet is a necessity; however, it is often ignored. Remember, 90 percent of the fatalities in bicycling are due to head injuries. Buy a helmet and WEAR it. "See and be seen" should be the motto of the safety conscious bicyclist.

PHYSICAL REQUIREMENTS OF THE ACTIVITY

There are no predetermined levels of endurance, leg strength, or conditioning that one must have before bicycling. This fact is one reason why it is so popular. However, as in any physical activity, the chance of injury increases with the onset of fatigue. Before mounting a bicycle, the bicyclist should be both physically and mentally alert, as both conditions contribute to the overall safety of the ride. Also, know your limits and quit bicycling when you become too fatigued.

COMPETITIVE CYCLING

Although the catastrophic injuries occurring in competitive cycling are no different than those found in recreational cycling, the situational stressors are different. Competitive cyclists usually train harder and "push themselves" nearer their physiological limits than do recreational cyclists. Crowds and superior opponents influence the physical and mental responses of the competitors and alter their performances. Greater risk-taking or greater fatigue may result in greater potential for catastrophic injury.

Impacts caused by crashes between riders during competition are primarily due to: 1)carelessness, 2)lack of experience, 3)fatigue, or 4)not wearing hard helmets.

Experienced riders usually know how to fall. They "bunch up" and take the fall with the muscular parts of their body, thus avoiding limb and head contact. Practice in falling from bicycles onto soft mats should be a part of the training regime of competitive cyclists. Strategies for passing other riders and potential danger situations must be taught. The riders must learn to recognize signs of fatigue, both mental and physical.

The use of hard hats and eye protection during practice and competition is advocated if the state-of-the-art equipment insures that vision, including peripheral vision, is not obscured and that the auditory sense is not reduced. Riders whose eyes are irritated due to insects, gravel, dirt, or other foreign objects striking the eye, should not wear a patch and continue to ride. Such coverage of an eye increases the risk of catastrophic injury.

When training or racing in hot weather, cyclists shall drink 13 to 20 ounces of fluid 15 minutes prior to riding and drink several ounces of fluid every 10 to 15 minutes during the ride (Burke 1986) to avoid dehydration. Diabetic riders having insulin-dependencies must be responsible for their own actions. They should have their medical remedies readily available and be aware of symptoms of need. They should inform team members and coaches of their medical problems.

The dangers of drugs, blood doping, and other such practices must be presented by the coach to all team members. Such practices have been suspected factors in deaths during long rides.

17

Boxing

Essam E.A. Moustafa
Helwan University, Alexandria, Egypt
Visiting, University of Illinois at Urbana-Champaign

For thousands of years, boxing has been one of the most popular combat sports. Boxing competition is a struggle between two boxers who have equal weight and experience. Every boxer tries to use skill to perform the boxing offense and defense strategies to win the competition within the boxing rules and the spirit of the rules.

Boxing, like other sports, has suffered through bleak periods and enjoyed boom periods, mainly due to increases and decreases in injuries occuring during competition. Whatever its temporary fortunes may have been, boxing has always survived because, historically, there always have been young men eager to meet the ultimate challenge in skill, strength, and cunning that boxing provides. The protests about boxing should encourage us to find better ways to prevent serious injuries and deaths (Table 17-1) instead of succumbing to the shouts to outlaw the sport.

POSSIBLE CATASTROPHIC INJURIES IN BOXING

Of course, there is no sport entirely without risk of injury. Moreover, there are few catastrophic injuries in boxing compared to some other sports. Boxing injuries rank eighth in frequency among sports injuries (Blonstein 1964). Statistics to support this statement are found in a report from the U.S. Consumer Products Safety Commission (CPSC) (Southmayer and Hoffman 1981) in which there was a listing of the number of sports injuries in more than 40 sports. From this report, we can make a comparison between boxing injuries and those of other popular sports.

Table 17-2 includes a listing of injuries in 10 sports in 1979, according to the CPSC. The injury data in boxing are not unique to that sport.

Table 17-1. Possible Catastrophic Injuries in Boxing

Activity	Possible Injury	Causes	Prevention
On guard (funda-mental position)	Concussion, Damage to brain, Fractures, Broken nose, jaw, teeth, Cuts around eyes, Abdominal injuries	Lack of good con-dition, Lack of technique training, Lack of sparring, Lack of proper pro-tective equipment	Keep in good physical condition. Learn proper tech-nique. Use protec-tive equipment, i.e., headguard, mouth-piece, cup. Keep equipment in good condition
Punching	Same as above plus fracture of thumb, metacarpals, elbow, and ankle	Same as above plus lack of competition	Same as above
Strategy	Same as above	Same as above	Same as above
Sparring without safety equipment	Any of the above-mentioned injuries	Poor timing and distancing of tech-nique, Lack of con-trol, Carelessness	Required use of safety equipment

Table 17-2. Total Number of Injuries in 10 Sports in 1979 and the Number and Percent of Injuries with Respect to Four Areas of the Body (CPSC 1979)

Sport	Total No. of Injuries	Face, Mouth, Eye, Ear		Shoulder		Head		Hand	
		Total	%	Total	%	Total	%	Total	%
Boxing	24,400	2,200	9.0	500	2.0	400	1.6	1,200	4.9
Bicycling	1,677,000	115,300	6.9	30,400	1.8	73,800	4.4	20,400	1.2
Track & Field	75,500	1,000	1.3	1,700	2.3	600	0.8	500	0.7
Wrestling	210,000	6,200	2.9	9,000	4.3	2,800	1.3	2,500	1.9
Rugby	26,100	3,300	12.6	1,200	4.6	700	2.7	400	1.5
Football	1,370,900	34,700	2.5	41,600	3.0	17,900	1.3	20,800	1.5
Soccer	270,300	7,300	2.7	2,400	0.9	4,000	1.5	1,900	0.7
Hockey	137,400	15,900	11.6	3,400	2.5	1,400	1.0	2,400	1.7
Volleyball	262,700	3,500	1.3	1,800	0.7	1,000	0.4	2,600	1.0
Basketball	1,292,000	36,100	2.8	8,500	0.7	8,900	0.7	10,300	0.8

Injuries to the face, mouth, eye, and ear are less than 10 percent of the total number of injuries. Hand injuries represent less than 5 percent of all injuries, and head injuries rarely happen (1.6 percent).

To reiterate, catastrophic injuries in boxing are not common. How-ever, the potential for serious injury exists and must be considered.

In boxing, the main target of attack, the hands, are the common sites of injury. It is evident that head injuries are the most serious catastrophic injuries in boxing. When a fighter sustains a blow to the head, the head is accelerated backwards or jerked. The brain, which is suspended in a cerebrospinal fluid inside the skull, will move the same way. The two main areas of the brain, gray and white matter, are accelerated, too, but at different rates. This difference in rate leads to shearing forces between the gray and white matter. Thus, some nerve cells can be damaged, and others can die, never to be replaced. Another thing that may happen in the collision of the brain with the skull itself is that in a frontal blow, both the front and back of the brain can be damaged. The common clinical presentation of this type injury is the individual who appears to be in a stupor or drunk. There is loss of memory related to time and place as well as loss of functional ability. A primary concern related to these clinical signs is that the boxer could have suffered a ruptured blood vessel. Bleeding will occur, leading to pressure on the brain, which may cause death (McLatchie 1984).

When a boxer has suffered a severe head injury, the world is informed. However, head injuries are not the most common type of injury to a boxer. This is borne out by the results of medical reports of three European Amateur Boxing Championships in which 508 boxers participated (Rome 1967; Miscole 1970; and Madrid 1971). With respect to the number of boxers participating, cuts were the most common injury, occurring in less than 8 percent of all boxers. These cuts were over or around the left or the right eye at the forehead. Of this number, less than 0.5 percent were severe enough to stop the bout.

Fractures to the thumb or metacarpal were the most common fracture-type injuries (less than 2 percent of the boxers). The nose was fractured in 0.5 percent of the boxers and fracture of the jaw or the ribs occurred with 0.2 percent of the boxers.

The referee stopped the contest in 12 percent of the contests to prevent any of the boxers from being badly injured. Four percent of the stoppages were in the first round, 5 percent in the second round, and 3 percent were in the third round.

During these competitions, less than 3 percent of the boxers were knocked out (KO). Of this group, 0.5 percent experienced the KO in the first round, 1.0 percent in the second round, and 0.5 percent in the third and last round. In none of these situations were the boxers unconscious more than 20 seconds (*The Journal of Sports Medicine and Physical Fitness*, Vol. 7, No. 4, and Vol. 11, No. 2 and 4).

PREVENTION OF CATASTROPHIC INJURY

Boxers should be given warning of dangers in boxing and what constitutes dangerous behavior.

1. The referee must know and enforce the rules. The referee must

recognize and decide when the boxer is hurt and when to step in immediately and stop the fight.

2. The important role of the coach to protect the health and safety of boxers cannot be minimized.

Physical Requirement of the Activity

As with most combative sports, it is necessary for boxers to be in top physical condition. Boxing requires a solid foundation to sustain hard knocks and to be able to respond with explosive power. The boxer's fitness could be the deciding factor to achieve a great degree of success in the ring. A high level of fitness will keep the boxer from getting tired and discouraged. It will allow the boxer to improve techniques and tactics rapidly in order to prevent catastrophic injuries.

The boxer needs muscular and cardiovascular endurance and flexibility in order to withstand fatigue, hardship, and stress through a strenuous competition. In amateur boxing, the boxer must fight nine minutes out of 11, getting only a minute's rest between each of the rounds of a three-round bout.

Throughout the competition, the boxer must throw the punches to the exact target in proper timing with suitable effective offense and defense strategy. Power, endurance, flexibility, coordination, agility, reaction time, and good body mechanics are recurring factors in the boxer's being able to win or lose the competition.

The boxer can increase physical fitness by skipping rope, roadwork, using medicine balls, speed bags, sand bags, shadow boxing, and sparring. Interval training, especially that which stimulates the tempo and rhythm of the competition, is the best method for increasing the boxer's conditioning level.

There is no doubt that the better the condition of the boxer, the greater the body control, thus, the lesser possibility of injury.

Proper Technique to Avoid Injury

The boxer must assume the on-guard position, which is the safest to allow complete relaxation of all muscles not involved in the action. At the same time, this gives maximum tension in the action muscles which is most favorable to quick reaction time. Proper technique helps to coordinate hands and feet so that maximum speed and efficiency will result, which, in turn, permit the greatest possibilities for either attack or defense. Boxing technique ensures that the feet are always under the body and, therefore, the body is always in balance. Actually, there are two times when the boxer is most likely to get hurt: either coming into the attack, or going away from the attack. For both situations, the boxer must return to the on-guard position with all possible speed after any offense or defense.

The boxer must continue to keep moving, as standing still invariably will result in being hit. However, the boxer must not waste energy by jumping around or making unnecessary movements. Boxer tactics include leading the opponent to puzzle him by a variety of movements. The boxer must punch the moment the opponent is in range and be aggressive with skilled punch combinations or the boxer will be placed on the defensive. The safest technique will be assured when the punch combinations are accurate and land on the correct target. Nothing is more important to a boxer than mastering the fundamental punches. The greater the mastery, the greater will be the possibility of winning the fight with safety, efficiency, and effectiveness.

In summary, when boxing is officiated and coached with the athlete's ultimate safety in mind, it is an art form of the highest order—the challenge of skill, strength, and cunning.

Boxing Equipment

Boxing equipment is used to protect the boxer from harm, reducing the risk of injury. Misuse, faulty, or improper design could be the main factor in causing injury. For this reason, boxing equipment must be carefully used and checked to make sure there are no imperfections before it is used again. A minimal amount of safety equipment is required for boxing.

The coach and the boxer must insist on wearing a properly padded headguard while sparring to absorb the effect of the shock of the punches on the boxer's brain to prevent catastrophic head injury.

The boxer should use a fitted rubber gum protector (mouthpiece) to decrease the impact of the punches on the face, to protect the mouth (teeth, gums, and jaws), and also to help protect the brain against this strong punch by reducing the transmission of force from jaw to brain.

The boxer must wear a proper supporter (cup) to protect against illegal punches from the opponent as well as blows from the opponent's knee on other body parts. Also, high-top boxing shoes are better protection against ankle injuries.

Another important part of boxing equipment is the gloves. The hand is not structured to be used as a dangerous weapon. However, once padded by gauze wrap and a 10-ounce leather glove, it could become a lethal weapon. The design of the glove therefore, should not only be engineered to protect the fighter's hand, but the opponent as well. For example, a leather shell with a minimum of polyurethane padding would protect the hand adequately, and at the same time, spread the shock of the blow over a wider area, preventing injuries due to blunt trauma.

The boxing ring should be properly maintained for the safety of the boxers. The ring floor must be checked for safety conditions. The ropes must be covered and tied, and the corners must have protective pillows. These conditions are to be met at all times, whether during training or competition purposes. Coaches and boxers must make sure that this protective equipment is kept in good condition and that suitable equipment is used in training and competition.

Boxing equipment should be examined before and after use to be sure it is free from any defects which could cause injury. Adequate storage must be provided for equipment when it is not in use. This will help protect boxing equipment and keep it safe from misuse, therefore decreasing the chance for unnecessary injuries.

RULES OF BOXING

The rules of boxing are based upon the knowledge that the effects of sustaining many minor head injuries over the years can accumulate. When this was recognized, there was public criticism of boxing and attempts were made to ban boxing. The result is that now boxing is probably one of the best medically controlled sports. There have been considerable reductions in the number of serious head injuries. Still, further attempts are being made to make boxing safer. There are many rules to follow, from the medical aspect, in order to protect the boxer from catastrophic injuries.

The major rules of safety are as follows:
1. The boxer must have a general diagnostic medical examination to determine level of physical fitness for boxing before beginning training.
2. Immunization must be given before boxers are allowed to compete in another country.
3. A Physician's examination must be given directly before going to weigh-in for any competition.
4. Boxers are prohibited from taking any drug before or during competition to protect them from any unnatural effects which would make them lose control of their bodies.
5. The competition cannot begin unless a physician is present to give medical attention immediately.
6. A boxer must take a rest from sparring or competition for a period of four weeks after sustaining a punch to the head (KOH) that renders the boxer unconscious for 10 seconds or more, and not be permitted to box again without a required medical examination. The boxer must rest for six months after the second KOH, and one year after a third KOH. The boxer must be certified medically fit before returning to the ring.

FUTURE CONSIDERATIONS

It is evident that boxing rules are designed to reduce the chance of injury. There is some suggestion that the boxing rules could be changed in order to make the boxer more safe from catastrophic injuries. Research and experimentation may be of value for the following suggested rule changes:

1. The ringside physician must have absolute authority to stop the bout at any time to prohibit unnecessary punishment to either boxer.
2. The referee and the ringside physican should be constantly in touch to safeguard against any unnecessary physical damage.
3. Specialized medical examinations should be given to those who want to be referees or seconds for the boxer.
4. The boxer MUST wear: A) the headguard and gum shields to protect from brain damage, and B) the bandage to prevent injuries to the hand.
5. Regular medical examination of amateur boxers must include electroencephalography, as done with the professional boxer, especially after KOH.
6. Restriction of target area and increased absorption of force of impact must be required.

18

Fencing

ANNE KATHRYN KLINGER
Clatsop Community College
Astoria, Oregon

Most persons view fencing as a sport of a previous era, or equate it with Hollywood movies. This view is far from accurate. In the United States today more than 4,000 active and serious competitors enjoy the sport, and more than 10 times that number participate in high school, college, and city park recreation programs. Fencing's popularity is growing at an astonishing rate. With so many participants, fencing instruction is sometimes offered by coaches who do not have a thorough understanding of the potential catastrophic injuries that could occur in fencing (Table 18-1). The purpose of this chapter is to acquaint the beginning teacher and coach, and remind the seasoned coach, of potential injuries, and to suggest ways in which these catastrophic injuries could be avoided.

POSSIBLE CATASTROPHIC INJURIES

There are two primary areas where catastrophic injuries could occur in fencing. These areas are 1) the head and neck area, and 2) the area under the armpit of the weapon arm. Catastrophic injuries which have or could occur in these areas include 1) concussion, 2), loss of vision, 3) serious internal damage to body organs, and 4) death. Fortunately, fencing has had a low rate of catastrophic injuries, yet two deaths have occurred in fencing in recent times; both of these occurred in world class competition.

Injuries which have occurred in fencing were due to one or more of the following factors:
1. The head is left completely unprotected.
2. The mask falls off during the action.

Table 18-1. Possible Catastrophic Injuries in Fencing

Activity	Possible Injury	Cause	Prevention
Lunge to hit head (epee)	Cut, Catastrophic head or face injury	Penetration of mask, mask-bib, or bib-jacket interface	Strongly meshed mask, Correctly fit-ted mask, bib, and jacket, Correct hit technique
Fleché with body contact	Whiplash, Broken weapon injury	Rough fencing, Poor technique	Use correct fleché technique, Penal-ize rough fencing
Lunge to body	Cuts, Bruises, Abrasions to thorax and vital organs	Broken blades, Slashing move-ments, Hacking	Emphasize dis-tance, Hit with point, Use proper attire
Cuts to head (sabre)	Possible concus-sion	Poor technique, Brutal hit	Correct head pro-tection, Proper dis-tance and technique
Incorrect carry of blade	Loss of eye	Ignorance or dis-regard of proper method of blade carry	Teach proper method of blade carry
Fencing without mask	Loss of eye, cut to artery	Ignorance or dis-regard of danger	Insist masks be worn at all times

3. The mesh of the mask fails and is penetrated by the blade or part of the fencing equipment.
4. The mask-bib interface is penetrated.
5. The bib-jacket interface is penetrated.
6. The blade breaks and penetrates the clothing of the fencer.
7. The fencer uses faulty or dangerous technique.

INSTRUCTOR RESPONSIBILITY IN PREVENTING HEAD AND NECK INJURIES

Preventing injuries to either of these body sites is the dual responsi-bility of the instructor and the student. Students must be instructed from the first day of class that competitive fencing is entirely different from stage fencing, and that actors who take part in stage fights are extremely skilled "stunt" persons who have trained for this activity and are fighting from choreographed scripts. There is no choreographed script in competitive fencing, especially in the case of beginners, whose skills are limited and whose actions are likely to be erratic and somewhat unpredictable. The beginner should be taught the "golden rule" of fencing: "Never cross weapons without wearing a mask," and its corollary, "Never point a blade at a person's face." These simple rules will greatly reduce the risk of a facial or head injury. Additionally, fencers need to be taught how to carry weapons. Weapons should always be carried by the tip or grip, and never placed over the shoulder. The rule for safe carrying is that the tip of the weapon is always visible to the person carrying it.

Students should be taught that they are responsible for their partner's safety as well as their own. The partners should check each other for safe apparel whenever the on guard position is assumed. Safe apparel includes the following:

1. Well-fitted mask with strong mesh and sewn-in bib of at least two thicknesses of cloth. New masks have been designed which have a strap across the back that connects both sides of the mask so it cannot fall off. If the mask lacks these straps, it should be squeezed and pressed to fit the individual. Masks should be numbered and used by one individual only; do not permit students to use just any mask. Encourage the student to make the mask fit better by sewing or gluing foam in the appropriate places on the mask. Rusty or dented masks should be destroyed. All class masks should pass the punch test. The bib should be of plastic or heavy duck, and should present one unbroken surface. Extra material can be sewn inside the bib or the bib can be taped completely across the front of the mask at the interface. The bib must fit securely against the jacket, and flat against the chest to prevent a blade point from sliding up under the mask.

2. The jacket must cover both arms to below the wrist and fasten on the correct side or in the back. Never permit a fencer to wear a jacket that fastens on the weapon arm side, as a weapon could slide through the fastenings. The jacket must be securely fastened at the collar at all times, and must completely cover the throat and side of the neck that faces the partner. Do not permit a student to wear a jacket that does not meet these requirements.

3. A glove must be worn on the weapon hand. The glove must be long enough to contain the sleeve of the jacket so that a point cannot penetrate between the glove and the jacket and run up the arm.

4. Women fencers must wear breast protectors. These may be made of any rigid material, with metal or plastic being the most common. Women should modify their class jackets so that the chest protector pockets fit properly.

5. Beginners especially should use blades which bend easily. Stiff blades tend to break more easily and can cause greater injury if used incorrectly. The handle or grip of the blade is also important in controlling the blade. Beginners should use only French grips

and not the orthopedic grips sometimes used by highly skilled fencers.

6. Underarm protectors (plastrons) are mandated by the rules. The plastron must be made of at least two thicknesses of cloth and include a sleeve on the weapon arm which extends below the elbow. There must be no seam or opening in the armpit area of the weapon arm. Additionally, when fencing sabre, a leather protector should be worn on the elbow. The mask should also be modified for sabre fencing by adding a roll of leather or strip of foam to the top of the mask.

SKILL PROGRESSION

One of the most important safety precautions in fencing is making the touch or hit correctly. Brutal hits and cuts are prohibited by the rules. The correct progression for learning to hit is as follows:

1. Discussion of right-of-way. Call attention to straightening the arm completely before the hit is made. No jabbing is permitted. After the point contacts the target, the hand should relax and allow the wrist to rise slightly.
2. Have the student extend the arm and hit a wall target or hard surface. The student must judge the distance and the weapon must bend *up* at the center following the hit. Students cannot be permitted to fence with a foil which bends the wrong way. This is sometimes caused by a fencer using a weapon intended for the opposite hand, and sometimes by faulty technique, such as holding the grip too tightly. Figure 18-1 illustrates the correct method of foil bend.
3. Student extends arm, advances, hits target.
4. Student extends arm, lunges, hits target.
5. Student extends arm at target area of properly attired partner. Partner walks on point of blade. Student relaxes arm at point of contact.
6. Student extends arm, advances, hits partner.
7. Student extends arm, lunges, partner walks on point.
8. Student lunges and hits partner. Partner is warned not to permit

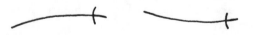

Correct   Incorrect

Figure 18-1. Correct foil bend method.

himself to be hit if the arm is not straightened before the lunge is executed, or if the arm is pulled back and then jabbed forward.

An important safety skill which must be mastered is the judging of distance. Misjudging or misuse of distance frequently causes broken blades, and broken blades can cause injury. The following skill progression and drills can be used in aiding the student in learning to judge distance.

1. Partners grasp opposite ends of a rope. As one advances, the other retreats. The object is to keep the same distance apart by keeping the rope taut.
2. Use the same drill, but one partner keeps the eyes closed and feels the distance by the pull of lack of pull on the rope.
3. Students pair off and keep distance from each other without weapons.
4. One student has a weapon, the other does not. The student without the weapon tries to keep the student with the weapon at the same distance from him by advancing and retreating.
5. Use the same drill, but both students now have weapons. One student acts as leader, and as such, is the only one who can use his weapon.
6. One student has a weapon and one does not. The student without the weapon sets the distance and the student with the weapon must extend the arm and advance, retreat, or lunge with the hit, depending on the distance set by the partner.

SPECIAL SAFETY CONSIDERATIONS

Equipment

Prior to every competition, a weapons and equipment check should be held. Any equipment that does not conform to the standards set in the USFA rulebook[1] should be confiscated for the duration of the competition.

Facilities

Fencing should not share space with any other activity, especially one involving balls. The floor used for fencing should be of wood or soft composition material. Rugs or foam mats can be used under regulation fencing strips to cushion shock. The strips for fencing must be laid out so that there is ample room for directors and judges to move freely up and down the sides of the strip without danger from the fencer's blades. There should be no obstructions at the end of the strips, and strips

---

1. *USFA Fencing Rules*, 1982 edition. USOC Training Center, Colorado Springs, Colorado.

should have at least 10 feet of space between the end of the the strip and the wall. If raised strips are used, they should end in ramps and not steps.

Directing

Qualified directors who enforce the rules concerning body contact and unsafe fencing should be employed to direct at all levels. Directors should retain complete control over the fencers and their equipment and should penalize unsafe fencing immediately. At novice levels, directors should explain unsafe actions to fencers so that they will know what the consequences of their actions could be.

In summary, the final responsibility for safety lies with the individual. The responsibility of the instructor is to make the student aware of dangerous actions and the possible consequences which could result from them. The instructor also has the responsibility to provide the student with sound and safe fencing equipment, to inspect the facility for possible dangers and remove them if possible, to teach the rules of fencing, and to keep the students under control at all times.

19

Golf

JON CHRISTOPHER
Washington State University
Pullman, Washington

Coaches need to inform their players of the following possible catastrophic injuries: (1) death, (2) loss of sight, and (3) coma with varying degrees of paralysis (Table 19-1).

PREVENTION OF CATASTROPHIC INJURIES

Warning of Dangers

Coaches must stress that the most prevalent cause of catastrophic injury is positionary and that the equipment used by the golfer is the primary potential cause of catastrophic injury. A combination of the hardness of the golf ball and clubhead and the speed of these objects during performance creates an environment for potential injury.

Golfers need to be informed of the danger of a ricochet when playing a shot where an object is close to the intended line of flight. When this danger is presented, golfers should be instructed to aim a comfortable, safe distance from the object. The golfer should inform other golfers of the possibility of a ricochet so they may seek a safe location and be alert to the flight of the ball.

Another area of potential danger for catastrophic injury is being struck by lightning while playing or practicing golf. Metal spikes in the shoes and the metal in the club compound the potential danger. Golfers must eliminate or reduce their chances of being struck by lightning at the first sign of danger. If on the course, golfers should avoid touching the clubs and should take off spiked golf shoes. If golfers must remain on the course, they should keep away from hilltops, wire fences, isolated trees, and open space. They should seek shelter in the largest building

Table 19-1. Possible Catastrophic Injuries in Golf

Activity	Possible Injury	Causes	Prevention
Practice tee, Teeing off, Course play	Loss of sight, Coma, Death	Being struck by a club or ball	Alertness and instruction on standing in a safe location out of possible line of flight of the ball or a thrown club
Drills	Loss of sight, Coma, Death	Being struck by a club or ball	Practice and drills performed in organizational patterns where a ball hit or a club swung or thrown cannot hit another golfer
Ricochet	Loss of sight, Coma, Death	Being struck by a ball	Golfers making each other aware of possible ricochets so non-hitting golfers may seek a safe location. The golfer hitting the ball should be instructed to aim a comfortable safe distance from the object
Practice, Course play	Coma, Disability, Death	Being struck by lightning	If practicing, stop and assume the safest spot available. If on the course, separate yourself from your clubs, take off spiked shoes, and assume the safest spot available
Practice, Course play	Coma, Death	Heatstroke	Awareness of possibility. Drinking plenty of liquids. Wearing a cap. Cooling the head and body with water

available, lowest ground, or dense woods, or they should lie flat. If practicing, they should stop and assume the safest spot available.

Coaches need to caution golfers on hot days to be aware of heat stroke. Players should be informed to drink plenty of liquids, wear a cap, and to cool the head and body with water.

Coaches also need to inform their players that in damp or wet weather they need to check the grip of the club and wipe it dry if needed before using.

Proper Instruction and Correct Technique

Coaches need to stress not only the importance of yelling a warning of "fore" to another golfer who is in danger, but also to instruct their golfers that when they hear such a warning they turn quickly and directly away from the direction of the warning, bending over slightly and covering their heads with their arms and hands. The judges in courts of justice agree that a warning shout is proper, but it should be made prior to the swing.

Coaches need to give instructions as to: where golfers should stand when another golfer is hitting, possible angles of flight a ball could travel, proper playing procedures emphasizing alertness when other golfers are hitting, and standing in a safe location.

Coaches need to use safe organizational patterns for practice and drills. Golfers should be arranged in lines so that balls or clubs cannot strike other golfers. During practice, golfers need to be instructed that they must never go ahead of the hitting line to retrieve a ball or club. Golfers should be instructed not to walk or step within the swinging distance of another golfer. Coaches should stress to their golfers that they should never stand in a location where a club that slips out of another golfer's hands or a ball hit on an unusual angle can strike them.

Coaches, when constructing practice situations such as chipping, pitching, and sand trap play, must provide adequate distance between golfers, so that if by reaction they move a step or two, they would not be in danger of being hit by a club or ball.

SPECIAL SAFETY CONSIDERATIONS

Rules and Etiquette for Safety

Golf is a game in which adherence to rules of courtesy and etiquette are essential for the purpose of the safety of others.

A major etiquette emphasis is that golfers are instructed to yell a warning of "fore" before they hit a ball that has a chance of striking another golfer. Other points of etiquette include: 1) the person furthest from the hole should hit first, and the playing partners should be in positions where there is no possibility of being hit by the club or ball; 2) a golfer should never hit a ball when it has a chance of striking a golfer in another group that is playing ahead; 3) once the group playing ahead has holed out, the next group must not hit until the group ahead is a safe distance from the green; 4) golfers are to record their scores on the tee of the next hole so they do not place themselves in a dangerous situation by staying around the green once they have holed out; 5) golfers should place their clubs hole high or to the back of the green in the direction of the next hole so that they will not be walking to the front of the green once they have holed out; and 6) throwing of clubs cannot be tolerated, not only because it is improper behavior, but also because of the potential danger of causing injury.

Facilities and Equipment

The design of golf courses gives primary consideration to safety in laying out holes to eliminate or reduce as much as possible conditions where a person playing another hole can be struck by the ball of another golfer. Players should play the course according to its design.

If clubs are provided for practicing or rental, they should be inspected periodically, and checked for cracks or breaks that could be dangerous. Records should be maintained noting the date of inspection and removal or repair of faulty clubs. Coaches should also have their golfers check their own clubs for cracks or breaks.

20

Gymnastics

BOB PEAVY
Washington State University
Pullman, Washington

MARLENE ADRIAN
University of Illinois at Urbana-Champaign
Urbana-Champaign, Illinois

Gymnastics activities have an unwarranted reputation as being hazardous. A recent study concluded that the number of severe injuries in organized gymnastics is low compared to other sports, and that fatal accidents are rare. However, death, paraplegia, and quadriplegia have occurred (Table 20-1), and the United States Gymnastics Federation (USGF) has launched a safety program.

Difficult, fast-moving routines, often performed in the air or on elevated equipment, have helped foster the idea gymnastics is dangerous. It can be. On the other hand, no less than three falls from loss of grip on a bar or missing the catch occurred at the 1986 Goodwill Games, and not a single gymnast was injured.

Brown and Wardell found that a number of factors—primarily negligence and unsafe equipment—can contribute to potential injury. Other factors cited included: improper warm-up, horseplay, attempting skills beyond ability, lack of or poor spotting, improper instruction, and unsafe environment. Monitoring such situations is essential in preventing catastrophic injury or death and subsequent legal actions. The United States Gymnastics Safety Association has been doing so since 1978 (Christensen and Clarke 1983).

WARNINGS

Head, neck, and back injuries in gymnastics usually result from falls. The primary concern of coaches and gymnasts is to understand all

Table 20-1. Possible Catastrophic Injuries in Gymnastics

Activity	Possible Injury	Cause	Prevention
Any skill on apparatus or floor exercise mat	Concussion, Paraplegia, Quadriplegia, Death	Falling	Proper skill progression. Concentrate. Stop prior to fatigue. Proper friction on hands. Optimum mat type and dimensions
Any skill on apparatus or on floor or exercise mat	Concussion, Paraplegia, Quadriplegia, Death	Equipment breaks, Spacing, Cracks on mats	Maintenance of equipment. Regular inspection of equipment. Landing training
Collision of performer and another gymnast	Concussion, Paraplegia, Quadriplegia, Death	Too many gymnasts for space, Disorganization of movement from station to station	Awareness of other performers. Policies for rotation among stations

the possible causes for falling and take precautions to prevent falls. The secondary concern is to manipulate the fall should one occur.

USGF has printed three safety posters recommended for display in the gymnastics training room. The two implicit warning statements forming the basis for these posters appear below.

1. "Catastrophic injury, paralysis, or even death can result from improper conduct of the activity."
2. "No gymnastic mat is a fail-safe to injury. Never land on the head, neck, or back on any type of mat, as serious, catastrophic injury, even death, could result."

PREVENTION

Prevention of catastrophic injuries is the responsibility of the teacher/coach and the gymnast. The teacher/coach must provide:

1. Competent supervision
2. Discipline and safe practice policies
3. Proper skill progression
4. Skill in responding to potential medical emergencies
5. Safe equipment, teaching devices, and adequate spotters

The gymnast has 10 responsibilities, according to the USGF Safety and Education Department.

1. Appreciation of risk
2. Practice only when supervised
3. **Dress appropriately**

4. Double check equipment
5. Communicate clearly
6. Be prepared to participate mentally
7. Master the basic skills first
8. Know the skill before attempting it physically
9. Always complete the action
10. Know self-limitations

The third important prevention and reduction of injuries lies in the area of safety guidelines for gymnastics mats. The rules for gymnastics competition include specifications for mats for specific uses. In general, safe use of mats includes the following:

1. Appreciation of performance limits of mats
2. Choosing appropriate mat for intended purpose
3. Inspection of mats regularly and maintaining constant vigilance.
4. Following manufacturer's guidelines

INSTRUCTION

The key phrase in teaching gymnastics skills is SAFETY AWARENESS. Gymnasts must think safety constantly. Total concentration must be encouraged during the learning stages and performances. The teaching of kinesthesis (body awareness) and balanced, safe landings will make up the majority of instruction. Some important teaching concepts are described in the next sections.

HORIZONTAL BAR AND UNEVEN PARALLEL BARS

These apparatuses can be dangerous to the gymnast because of the their heights. An unexpected fall could contribute to serious injury. The 1985 edition of the *USGF Gymnastics Safety Manual* recommends that mats or pads of specific minimum size and thickness to prevent shock and eliminate injury be placed under the apparatuses and in the landing area.

While gymnasts perform on the horizontal bar and uneven parallel bars, centrifugal force often pulls them away from the apparatuses. If the force is too great to counteract, the gymnasts involuntarily release their grips.

Taylor showed most accidents on the horizontal bar result from: 1) the body arching during the first part of the routine when the head is thrust backwards on regular grip giant circles; 2) the complete movement is performed in a bent body position, usually characterized by a small angle between the arms and body; and 3) the body stretching too soon or too late during the second part of the circle.

Precautions should be taken to correct technical faults leading to involuntary release immediately after completing the downward swing.

Other deficiencies in long and short body swings are related to incomplete rotation, elliptical swing, and sideward swing.

Incomplete rotation is usually attributed to insufficient velocity and the loss of potential to rise. To avert danger, the athlete should switch immediately to a mixed hand grip and shorten the radius of the swing as quickly and completely as possible. Next, the gymnast must bend the arms, bend at the waist, and roll the wrists toward the apparatus. At or just beyond the low point of the swing, the gymnast should be prepared to receive a jerking action.

Elliptical swings can be prevented on a bar if the athlete remains fully extended through the bottom vertical phase of the swing and uses a pike of the shoulders on the upward phase. Too much speed can develop in one phase of an elliptical circle, which makes the maneuver difficult to control.

Athletes should develop strength equally in both arms. Sideward swing usually occurs when an athlete fails to push the body away from the apparatus symmetrically with both arms. If one arm fails to extend itself equally with the other, the body will swing sideward outside the plane of the hands, arms, and shoulders, usually resulting in loss of control of swing and release from bar.

Bower states faulty posture—arching, sagging, or loose hips—induces loss of control. In such cases, athletes should be instructed to cease activity immediately or be stopped by a spotter.

According to Miki, learning basic swing on the horizontal bar is the most important safety consideration. He suggests the following techniques:

1. Hand push the bar straight upward at the vertical point on any swing.
2. Develop the strength to make proper positions.
3. Keep arms straight at all times.
4. Tightness of the body is an important factor in developing a correct action.
5. Extension of the body is essential for making smooth and large swings.

RINGS

Height and swing movement can contribute to serious injury. When traditional swing movements (such as dislocate, inlocate, front and back giant circles) are performed, the gymnast may involuntarily be forced to release one or both hands. The gymnast should try to keep constant pressure on the rings and push the body away from the apparatus on the downward swing. The gymnast should lead with the chest rather than allow the feet to fall first. If the feet drop too quickly, the body will be jerked from the rings at a point just beyond vertical at the bottom of the swing. Active spotting of dislocates, inlocates, and giant circles in either direction is encouraged until the athlete develops a smooth, fluid swing and feels confident enough to perform the maneuver alone.

FLOOR EXERCISE, VAULTING, BEAM, AND DISMOUNTS

One of the most common causes of injuries in gymnastics stems from incorrect somersaults. Multiple somersaults, with or without twists and in different directions, are common in higher levels of gymnastics. Coaches and athletes should be careful to prevent uncontrolled landings on head, neck, or back. Proper lead-ups should be stressed so athletes will be familiar with their position in the air relative to landing mats.

Disorientation is another problem for gymnasts. Practicing a maneuver many times helps develop awareness in somersaulting. In multiple somersaults, a competent spotter should be present. It is imperative that athletes keep their eyes open throughout maneuvers to locate the mat before landing.

Under or over rotation of aerial somersaults can cause improper landings on the balance beam and unpredictable falls. Repetition of potentially dangerous maneuvers should be first practiced at a suitable height. Coaches and gymnasts should proceed with caution when learning difficult moves—with special consideration being given for age, weight, condition, experience, and ability of the athlete.

CERTIFICATION

Gymnastics coaches and teachers are encouraged to affiliate with the USGF, enroll in its safety certification program, and become certified. The USGF offices are located at 1099 N. Meridian, Suite 280, Indianapolis, Indiana 46204.

21

Handball

ROGER C. WILEY
Washington State University
Pullman, Washington

In the early 1900s, handball began as an intercity game for eastern city youth and young adults. Its popularity quickly spread from the one-wall game to the present day four-wall court game. It is one of the truly "bilateral" games in our socity with equal skill being demanded of either hand. While originally designed for boys and men, the game can be and is played by girls and women.

For individuals who make their livelihoods primarily with their hands, (such as surgeons, dentists, architects, and muscians) special care must be given to the protection and care of the hands and arms. For all players of handball, *special care must be given to the protection of the eyes.*

POTENTIAL CATASTROPHIC INJURIES

1. The loss or impairment of vision due to being struck in the eye by the ball or by the hand or another player.
2. Disability of the hand or upper arm as a result of hitting the wall with an open hand or clenched fist.
3. Brain injury which results from a blow to the head due to contact with another player or contact with the front or back wall, floor, or open door.
4. Dehydration or heatstroke which result from extended play when the court is *extremely warm* and/or has poor ventilation.

PREVENTION OF CATASTROPHIC INJURY

Handball, as compared to racquetball, brings the player in closer contact with the opponents and with the wall surfaces. Often players are struck by the hitting player on the back swing or follow-through. Special instructions regarding appropriate spacing are to be given early in formal instruction. In warning of possible dangers inherent in handball play, all participants, from the beginning to the more advanced players, should be instructed in the following:

1. Eye injuries—Injuries to the eyes are one of the most common types of injury, and eye or glass guards must be worn AT ALL TIMES. At no time, should a player enter a handball court without eye protection of some kind. Guards that are worn must meet American Society of Testing and Materials (ASTM) specifications. Additional information is provided in Chapter 24.

2. Collision Possibilities—A thorough knowledge of the game and its rules is essential. It is usually necessary to demonstrate to beginning players an actual singles and doubles game with specific information being given on those phases of the game where players *negotiate* for space and danger of collision is greatest.

3. Watch the Ball—Following the flight of the ball is very important since much of the game is dependent upon knowing the location of the ball and the position of opponent(s) on the court. Players must be able to anticipate the moves of opponents and thus plan their counter-moves with safety as a factor of importance. While it is natural to watch the path of the ball at all times, if one is in front of the ball while it is being played by an opponent, a player *must not turn around* to see where the ball has gone or what the opponent may do with the return.

4. Hand and Arm Injuries—One of the common injuries to the hands and arms in handball occurs when players strike the wall accidentally. This can result in a finger sprain or a dislocation or fracture of the hand, arm, or shoulder. In playing a ball that is close to the wall (hugging the wall), extreme care must be taken when hitting the ball with a sidearm stroke. Body alignment in these situations is important, as is arm stroke. An overhead stroke or underhand stroke is much preferred in such situations.

5. Position on Court—Players should be cautioned to be aware of their position on the court. Diving or running into walls in an attempt to play a ball is dangerous and can result in severe injury. In the course of play, players should move out of the back court in order that opponents attempting to retrieve a ceiling ball or backwall ball can avoid a collision. *It is the responsibility of the player who has just made a shot to get out of the way of an opponent.*

6. Condition of the Ball—During play, and especially on the service, every effort must be made to keep the ball dry. A wet ball slides unpredictably off the court surfaces, resulting in unplanned or out of control movements and injury. In the event

that the gloves become wet, a dry pair must be substituted. It is the responsibility of the *server* to check the condition of the ball.

7. Player Condition—Poor conditioning can lead to excessive fatigue. This in turn can lead to less player mobility and inappropriate court position. It can also lead to loss of control of the body and can increase the chance of falling or striking another player or the court surfaces. Every session of play should be preceded by a warm-up of the upper and lower extremities, especially the arms, hands, and shoulders.

8. Court Conditions—Temperature and humidity are conditions that must be monitored—any time the humidity is greater than 70 percent and the temperature is more than 80 degrees Fahrenheit, water breaks and periods of rest must be scheduled. It is usually wise to take rest breaks after every game and, if needed, periodically during a game.

9. Court Entrance—General court construction consists of doors that are lower than normal. Players must be careful coming and going and must knock before entering a court, determining first that play has stopped. An unannounced entrance increases the possibility of being struck by a player or the ball. Also, it adds the possibility of a player running into an open door.

Three areas of concern are always paramount: a) equipment is safe and appropriate; 6) participants are properly conditioned; and c) each session of handball is conducted with skills that are built on previous skills and are progressively more difficult in order to ensure safe play.

THE CORRECT TECHNIQUE TO AVOID INJURY

The causes of injury in handball are usually improper hand care, improper use of stroke in playing shots near the walls, or reckless play in charging after balls. Many times injury can be avoided if players practice courtesies common to good handball etiquette. It is usually wise that only players of comparable skill play each other so that frustration does not lead to careless play.

One of the most exacting phases of play requiring high-level sportsmanship is the calling of *hinders*. It is generally considered appropriate if your opponent legitimately interfered with your shot, either by being too close to you or by obstructing your view of the ball, to call a hinder. Because of close quarters and the intimacy of play, all players must adhere to the highest ideals of handball sportsmanship.

"Fighting for the center of the court" is a strategy common in handball. That position, at the service line and midway between the walls, becomes important as one learns handball. Many times, this places the player in a position of being in front of a ball being played. In situations of this kind, it is "an unwritten rule" that one never turns about to face the rear of the court. Instead, a player faces the front of the court and depends upon peripheral vision and the sounds of the opponent and the ball to maintain a safe position on the court. As a player passes from the ranks of beginner to intermediate, the player learns to "peek" over a raised elbow and arm protecting the face and head and at the same time stealing a look at the play of the opponent.

Balls are constantly rebounding in a plane parallel to the side wall—many times so close that even the most skilled players cannot strike the ball without hitting the wall. In stroking such a ball, one must slide the hand along the wall either in an overhead or underhand sweeping motion. It is difficult for a beginner to anticipate a close "wall ball." When in doubt, it is usually wise to avoid possible injury by not attempting to strike the ball. The gain or loss of a point is usually not worth the injury caused by an improper swing.

A shot popular with many intermediate and advanced players is the clenched fist or "punch" shot. While used with a short jabbing action in mid court, it is usually not advisable that such a shot be used on backwall or sidewall play, especially when the ball is close to the wall.

A beginning player soon discovers that in the early phases of handball play, "toughness of the hands" causes the greatest concern. The hand is unaccustomed to striking the handball, and bone bruises and hand swelling are common. In the former, the exposed bony parts of the hand become discolored and extremely painful if play is continued. There are usually two recourses—the first is to discontinue play until the bone bruise disappears, and the second is to play with a sponge or padding in the glove. Continuing to play with bruised hands, which are untreated, can lead to careless play and more permanent injury to the hands.

Many beginners prefer to use a soft sponge in the hands in the early phases of learning, until the hands are conditioned. Soaking the hands in hot water before play and slapping the hands together during warm-ups is another technique commonly used to minimize swelling.

Next to the hands, handball players consider care of the feet to be of great importance. Because handball is a game of quick starts and constant lateral or forward/backward movement, many participants prefer to use two pair of socks to lessen discomfort to the feet. This practice usually prevents blisters caused by excessive foot movement within the shoe and may provide more stability during changes of direction by the player.

Warm-ups should start with calisthenics designed to stretch the muscles of the arms and legs and condition the connective tissue around the joints. Arm circles, side stretching, trunk bending and twisting, running in place, calf stretching (similar to that done by a jogger), and throwing the ball to the front wall with both arms are usually the types of exercises and drills used. Players should never begin a game of handball until they are well warmed up. It is sometimes wise for the players to play a five-point game at slow to medium speed to get the feel of the court, ball, and opponent(s), and then to progressively work into more strenuous play.

Progression Of Skills

Drills that teach court positioning, ball control, and shot placement and that go from simple skill to more complex play should be used. Initially players need to be able to learn the basic strokes of underhand, side arm, and overhand; the power, low drive, and lob serve; and side wall and rear wall play. Players should begin to utilize both hands early in the learning sequence. As the skill of the players increase, other skills of a complex nature should be added. These include such fundamentals as the diagonal or Z serves, kill, pass and ceiling shots, hop serves and returns, and front and corner shots and kills. As the players work on skill development, emphasis should be on development of hitting technique, moving on the court, placement of shots, and *appropriate positioning in relation to the opponents and the ball*

Physical Requirements of Handball

The better the physical condition of the player in handball, the less likely the chance of severe or catastrophic injury. Fatigue will increase the incidence of player contact and result in sloppy court and wall play.

SPECIAL SAFETY CONSIDERATION

Respect for the rules of handball, especially the hinder, will help players to avoid injury. When players block the path to the ball, do not charge—simply call a hinder. If you are close at the ball—injury to yourself, as well as to your opponent can be avoided.

Quite often, injury in handball can occur when the ball is not in play. Careless hitting of the ball to or at an opponent in a dead ball situation is inappropriate—always roll the ball to your opponent.

The game of doubles is potentially more dangerous to players than the game of singles or cut-throat. Court positioning should be stressed, and all players need to be aware of the location of the ball at all times. Quite often the development of understanding the "sounds of the ball" will assist players in appropriate court position and an anticipation of ball location.

Handball is an intense game with competitive action more severe than some other types of "dual games." The loss of temper can create, for all individuals, situations that increase the likelihood of injury. Instructors must not allow play when tempers replace sound and controlled play.

22

Judo

MICHAEL PURCELL
Richland, Washington

Judo is a sport of high impact and torsional forces. Considering that a prime objective of judo is for one competitor (judoka) to throw his or her opponent to the back, it is fortunate indeed that serious injuries to head and neck are rare.

Generally, such injuries cannot be attributed to particular technique; they are a function of fatigue leading to poor throws, partial blocks, and incomplete counters. Since the mid-1960s, however, the improper application of one style of seoinage (shoulder throw) has increased the incidence of injuries to the head and neck.

"Dropping seoinage" was introduced to American judo by the Japanese judoka Yasuhiko Nagatoshi who, at 154 pounds, won the United States National Grand Championship (all weights) in 1967. Nagatoshi's application of the throw was brilliant, and never the cause of injury, but his imitators were not so successful. In the properly executed throw, tori (the thrower) pivots and drops to a squat in front of uke (the receiver); the forward pull continues high over tori's head as the legs drive up and forward; only when uke is well off the mat does the pull curl down, snapping the opponent over (Figure 22-1). At no time during the throw does uke's head come within two feet of the mat.

Unfortunately, many judoka attempting the throw see only the pivot and drop, allowing their hands to follow the downward motion, pulling uke's head into the mat (Figure 22-2). Serious injuries have resulted.

PREVENTION

Head Protection Equipment

Helmets have never been seriously considered for judoka. As active as a judo match can be, a helmet would become a weapon, not a safety device.

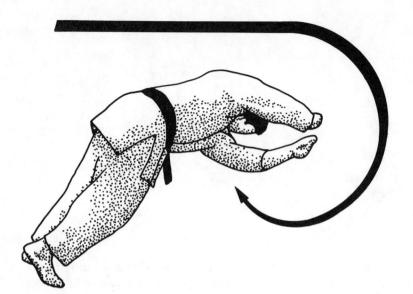

Figure 22-1. Properly executed throw.

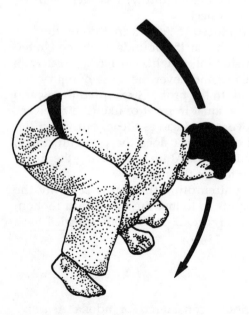

Figure 22-2. Improper throw.

The mat is, then, the only physical protection that can be offered a judoka. There are three mat surfaces in common use: traditional tatami (straw matting, now plastic coated), wrestling mats, and foam mats.

Tatami is a very fast, firm surface that itself provides little protection against concussion. Properly installed, tatami is mounted on a sprung floor or rollers that absorb sudden shock. Unfortunately, such mat mounting systems are rare in this country.

Wrestling mats are excellent protection against the kinds of major injuries caused by dropping seoinage, but their extreme softness and stickiness contribute to a high rate of less serious injuries to the toe, ankle, and knee.

Foam matting is an excellent compromise in firmness and protection. Since such matting is usually pieced together from four by eight feet or five by ten feet sections leaving gaps, a one-piece cover is essential for protection against toe and ankle injuries.

Falling Skills

All judoka must have excellent falling (ukemi) skills. Fear of falling is not only a grave safety hazard, but subtly undermines all aspects of throwing offense and defense.

Judoka usually thrust an arm out to prevent a throw's completion for one of two reasons: they have not overcome "natural" reflexes (inadequate physical training), or they have lost their competitive perspective to the point of self-injury (poor coaching). Broken arms, broken collarbones, dislocated elbows, and acromioclavicular dislocations are common results. With a driving, forward technique like dropping seoinage, the slowing of momentum resulting from judoka trying to "catch" themselves can contribute to even more serious injuries to head and neck.

Fortunately, it is rare to find judo training where competent ukemi instruction is not available. Care must be taken, however, to insure individual attention; each phase of the training *must* be mastered before moving to the next. Also, as students become advanced competitors, ukemi must not be eliminated from their training regimen. Rotation through throwing drills like numbers 2 and 4 below insure practice in this vital skill.

TECHNIQUE IMPROVEMENT

Drills:

1. **Uchikomi:** Uchikomi is the repetitive practice of a technique without throwing. Long a foundation of judo practice, its value remains undiminished. To be effective, uchikomi must be supervised by a knowledgeable coach; practicing an improper tech-

nique is counter-productive. Speed should be discouraged until technique execution is sound.

2. **Jumping Drill:** To emphasize the up and forward drive of the legs, have the judoka pivot and drop into the low loading position and then spring into a shoulder roll (on the right side if the seoinage is executed on the right side) *over* another judoka in a hands-and-knees position in front of him (Figure 22-3).

3. **Pulleys or belt-pull:** Using a pulley system or belt wrapped around a pole at chest height, pivot and drop into the loading position, pushing the hands forward as far as possible while keeping them well above the head (Figure 22-4).

4. **Throwing line:** Once the fundamentals of the throw have been mastered, there is no substitute for actual practice. The most time-efficient method involves having one tori repeatedly throwing many different uke in succession. This limits the number of falls any one uke receives, and allows tori to concentrate on small adjustments to the technique. Like uchikomi, this practice should be closely supervised, and speed never allowed to compromise the quality of the throw.

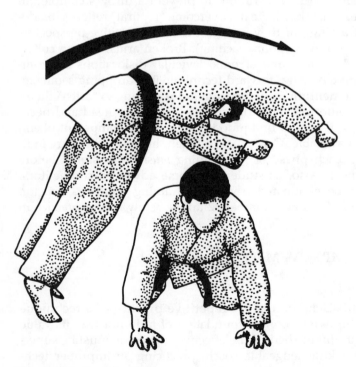

Figure 22-3. Jumping drill.

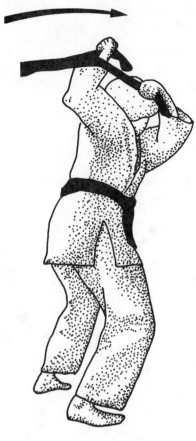

Figure 22-4. Belt pull.

While the drills listed above have proven helpful in developing a sound and safe technique, no amount of rote physical practice will replace the improvements seen when a judoka comes to understand the principles behind the throw: the dropping motion is only an extremely fast method for getting below uke's center of gravity, and the pull and leg drive must be forward, remaining high as long as possible.

23

Karate

MARGARET R. FRIMOTH
Karate for Women
Astoria, Oregon

Any martial art, by its very nature, is susceptible to catastrophic injuries. It is vitally important to recognize that contact sports can be dangerous, and to instill this knowledge in students. Karate ceases to be a viable learning experience when students spend most of their time wondering how they might get hurt.

In many ways, karate is first a discipline, and secondly, a physical regime. Taught with this in mind, karate will have virtually no catastrophic injuries. Too often, however, the preliminaries of instruction are skimmed over, sometimes skipped entirely, to encourage more participants in classes, to promote sparring (free-form fighting), and to accommodate classroom/class time scheduling. Beginning instruction is the critical learning time for students. Negligence or hurried exposure to beginning instruction will promote potential injuries (Table 23-1).

There is danger not only to the students of karate, but also to the karate instructors. Schmidt (1975) described three cases of fatal anterior chest trauma to karate instructors. Causes of death included aspiration and asphyxia, cardiac arrest, and traumatic rupture of the spleen. Failure to "pull" delivered techniques just short of anatomical impact was the primary mechanism responsible for death in all cases. It is suggested that instructors modify potentially hazardous training procedures in an effort to eliminate unnecessary fatal traumatic injury

POSSIBLE CATASTROPHIC INJURIES

The karate instructor teaches students to target at vulnerable body areas. Catastrophic injuries occur because of *improper, excessive, or uncontrolled contact* to any vulnerable body part (Figure 23-1). These injuries include blindness, concussions, skull fractures, ruptured ear drums,

Table 23-1. Possible Catastrophic Injuries in Karate

Activity	Possible Injury	Cause	Prevention
Hand/foot techniques to face and head area	Excessive abrasion and laceration to skin, Contusion, Blindness, Loss of teeth, Ruptured ear drum, Broken facial bones, Concussion, Death	Out of control technique, Misjudgment of distancing, Poor technique	Safety equipment, Enforced and focused control, Proper understanding of technique
Hand/foot techniques to vulnerable body targets	Excessive abrasion to skin, Ruptured internal organs, Broken ribs, Extreme damage to foot bones, Neck and spine damage, Death	Same as above	Same as above
Takedowns and sweeps	Head, neck, and spine damage, Broken bones, Injury to joints	Improper technique, Dropping or throwing opponent without control, Using force against joints	Proper and careful instruction of techniques, Slow practice, Use of ground pads during practice, Use of personal safety equipment
Sparring without safety equipment	Any of the above-mentioned injuries	Poor timing and distancing of technique, Lack of control, Carelessness	Required use of safety equipment

neck/spine injuries, kidney damage, lacerations (especially to the face and neck area), broken limbs or ribs, joint injury, damage to internal organs, injury to genital areas, and potential fatalities. Bruising from repeated technique practice is unavoidable. Jammed fingers and toes are probably unavoidable as well, although continuous attention given to proper technique will prevent these minor injuries from becoming major. Careful and exacting instruction will greatly reduce the number of injuries to the student.

Students learn proper target areas for defense in "real" fights. They must then distinguish those self-defense targets from acceptable target areas in karate sparring matches. It should be stressed that while sparring, no attack is ever exerted aginst a joint, particularly knees and ankles. The legs become vulnerable targets as a student increases in

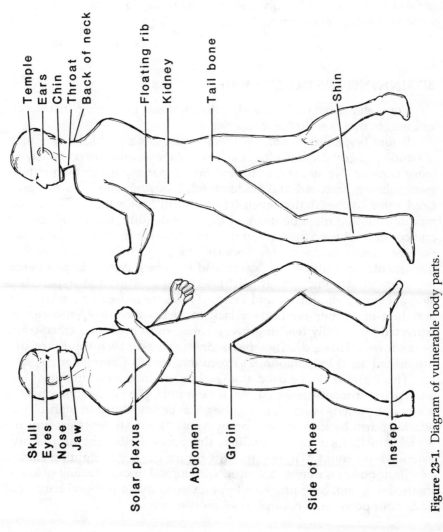

Skull
Eyes
Nose
Jaw

Solar plexus

Abdomen

Groin

Side of knee

Instep

Temple
Ears
Chin
Throat
Back of neck

Floating rib

Kidney

Tail bone

Shin

Figure 23-1. Diagram of vulnerable body parts.

skill, especially if she/he is learning any floor technique such as sweeps and takedowns. Whenever possible, sweeps and takedowns should be practiced on mats or other floor padding. Instructions should be as thorough as basic beginning lessons. Possibilities for catastrophic injuries double when floor techniques are used because of the potential for improper, excessive, or uncontrolled contact, AND the unexpected disastrous fall of the opponent. In karate, the attacker always assumes responsibility for an opponent's fall. Therefore, an attacker must remain in control of the sweep or takedown throughout the technique until the opponent is safely on the floor. It is imperative to impress upon students that performing a floor technique does *not*, in and of itself, score a point. The sweep or takedown must be followed with a controlled, appropriately targeted attack. Simply showing off skills does not score points. Control must be maintained.

BEGINNING INSTRUCTION

Competent, controlled, and individualized beginning instruction will negate most catastrophic injuries.

Before beginning to spar, students must understand the essentials of hand/eye/body coordination, balanced stances, and correct attack/defense motions. Never send a student into a sparring match before these essentials are practiced and understood. Sparring usually is not practiced prior to the sixth, seventh, or eighth lesson hour. The initial month's training must be devoted to understanding technique, power, and control. Without this critical time for students to develop their abilities, problems are inevitable because sloppy technique, uncontrolled movements, and misuse of power lead to almost certain impairments.

Non-catastrophic though distressing injuries include hyperextension of elbows, shoulders, and knees. These are caused by a misunderstanding of proper method or lack of focused control, and can be corrected by initially teaching every karate movement in a three-count breakdown. Three distinct parts of each basic technique are distinguished as: 1) Preparation, 2) Execution, and 3) Completion.

This formula can be used as a teaching method by counting, "One" and having students demonstrate, for example, the preparation phase of a straight punch—step from fighting stance into forward stance, pull attacking arm back to waist; during count "Two" students execute the actual punch, focusing (or pulling) the punch before the arm is fully extended; on count "Three" students return quickly to fighting stance.

Basic body awareness balanced with logical understanding of karate methodology not only prevents hyperextension and physical harm, but adds both power and control to all movements.

INSTRUCTING "CONTROL"

During the first month of lessons, prior to sparring, students can be paired off and directed to practice various basic attack and defense exercises. This teaches distancing and timing, and establishes the foundation for implementing control. Power and focused control can be taught in several different ways, one being to use padded targets or bags and ask students to practice each basic technique by hitting the target five times with as much power as possible while maintaining proper technique. Then, instruct students to use as much power and speed as they did previously, but to "pull" or stop the technique one fourth inch away from the pad. Once students understand and accomplish the control emphasized in this exercise, and once they have a basic repertoire of attacks and defenses, they are ready to begin sparring. It is advisable to initiate sparring with same-level beginning students, or to have beginning students spar with advanced students who are skilled in control and focus. After experiencing a few matches, students can be encouraged to spar with everyone (all levels) in the club, as often as possible to improve technique, detailed movement, and control.

SAFETY EQUIPMENT

Karate students are more prone to injury if safety equipment is *not* used. Many schools are suggesting that safety equipment is not necessary or that it is not as "real" as fighting without equipment. This "macho attitude" is simply karate jargon—a lingo that tends to promote undisciplined learning and dangerous power. When injury prevention is a precedent, the use of safety equipment is not an issue.

Protective, padded gloves, and foot coverings must be made available and required for sparring. Students should be required to purchase mouthguards. Male students must purchase groin cups. Both mouthguards and cups are usual mandatory items during tournament competition. Other protective padding that is advisable includes forearm, shin pads, knee, and elbow pads. Because repetition is regularly utilized during practices, padding eliminates many small, uncomfortable bruises, leaving more time for progressive learning. Ice or other cold pressure should be available for use on minor injuries.

Gloves and foot coverings are not necessary when performing Kata (individual forms). Gloves and foot coverings become cumbersome and awkward when one is developing more intricate patterns of movement and coordination. Knee and elbow pads may be worn if the student desires, particularly if drop kicks, falls, and/or rolls are used in the Kata.

24

Racquetball

MARY ANN BAYLESS
Elk River, Minnesota

Racquetball is a game played in a confined area with each player having a racquet and under circumstances which require that both (or all, in doubles or cut-throat) players move continually from one position to another in response to a fast-moving ball and in relation to another player. Being hit with the ball and/or an opponent's or one's own racquet are obvious threats. Anyone playing racquetball, and anyone coaching racquetball players, should be intensely aware of these conditions and the possibility of catastrophic injury (Table 24-1).

POSSIBLE CATASTROPHIC INJURIES

Catastrophic injuries related to racquetball include:
1. The loss of vision as a result of being struck in the eye by the ball or a racquet.
2. Brain injury resulting from a racquet blow to the head or from a blow to the head due to contact with a wall or fall to the floor.
3. Spinal injury, usually in the area of the fourth and fifth cervical vertebrae, as a result of contacting the wall head first, usually while moving to get a low shot.

PREVENTION OF CATASTROPHIC INJURY

Warning of Dangers and Dangerous Behavior

All participants, especially beginning players, should be instructed that:
1. Lack of knowledge or not using the structure of play intended for racquetball increases the chance of injury.
2. A ball striking the eye can cause permanent damage and loss of vision. Eye guards meeting American Society for Testing of Mate-

Table 24-1. Possible Catastrophic Injuries in Racquetball

Activity	Possible Injury	Cause	Prevention
Being struck by a racquet during rally	Head injury, Brain damage, Eye injury	Being struck by own racquet	Correct hitting technique
		Being struck by opponent's racquet	Playing correct court position in relation to the hitting player and shot being attempted
Being struck by the ball during a rally	Eye injury	Ball strikes fully on eye	Wearing adequate eye guards. Playing in correct position in relation to hitting player. Taking a correct "ready" position when the opponent is hitting
Running into the wall	Head injury, Neck injury	Striking the head on the wall	Not diving for a ball close to the wall. Knowing how to play a ball close to the wall. Playing in a correct position

rials (ASTM) specifications should be worn when playing. Eye guards which have an open space with no "lens" give some protection, but a direct hit can still result in the ball damaging the eye. This type of guard does not meet ASTM specifications.

3. A blow to the head resulting from a racquet or from running into a wall can cause severe injury and possible brain damage.
4. Causing "hinders" or not calling hinders puts a player in a position of possible injury.
5. Entering a court without knocking and determining that play in the court has stopped puts a player in a position of possible injury.
6. Hitting oneself with the racquet results from poor hitting technique. Correct body positioning when hitting is important to safe play.
7. Lack of conditioning leads to excessive fatigue. Fatigue results in less player mobility and increases the possibility of inappropriate court positioning, which in turn increases the possibility of being

struck by another player's racquet or the ball. Excessive fatigue also causes loss of control of body and increases the chances of falling or striking the head against the court surfaces or another player.

CORRECT TECHNIQUE TO AVOID INJURY

The cause of injury in racquetball is often the direct result of poor stroke technique: striking oneself with the racquet, striking oneself with the ball, or striking another player with an errant shot. The catastrophic injury danger in hitting oneself in the face with the racquet often occurs at the end of the swing after ball contact when a great amount of force has been generated. This can result in severe damage to an eye or the cranium. The racquet may be brought back into the body because of any number of errors which result in the post-contact swing of the racquet being limited in its path toward the front wall. This could include facing the front wall when hitting, hitting when the ball is too close to the body, or any other ball-body relationship which causes the performer to step away or shift the weight away from the ball during the hitting action.

If poor technique is used when hitting the ball into the back wall, the usual result is that the ball hits the back wall and rebounds, striking the hitter in the face. To avoid this situation, a player should anticipate the point at which the ball will be played into the back wall and play it either on the forehand or backhand side, as appropriate. The body should be positioned to the side of the ball, and the ball should be struck so that its flight toward the front wall (rebounding off the back wall) will not be into the hitter's body or face.

Controlling shots, so that the ball will travel to the desired point of aim, cannot be accomplished without the development of correct hitting technique. Players should be instructed in all facets of stroke execution, including grip, ready position, moving to the ball, setting up to hit, and the hitting action. Being able to control the direction of the ball contributes to the safety of play in two ways. First, it greatly reduces the chance that the opponent will be struck by an errant shot. Second, it allows for positioning and use of court space since the hitting player knows the area from which the opponent will be playing the next ball. This in turn alleviates crowding in the center court area, which is often the case when players cannot control shot placement.

Hitting strategically correct shots also contributes to a game that has a lower risk of anyone being struck by the ball or racquet. In order to take the front court position (center court), a player wants to force the opponent to play: 1) along the sides of the court and 2) deep in the court. This means that a player must learn to hit the ball accurately so that: 1) the ball travels along the walls without rebounding off the side wall into center court and 2) the ball travels into the back court without bouncing off the back wall. Accomplishing this allows the player to move into center court without being in the other player's way.

The predominant contributing factor to injury in racquetball is improper court positioning. The strategy of racquetball indicates that the center court area slightly behind the service area is advantageous. However, a player should not return a ball that is in play and then take a position in the center court area, regardless of the ball's flight path. Such action increases the likelihood of being struck by the ball or an opponent's racquet. COURT POSITION MUST BE ADJUSTED DEPENDING UPON THE FLIGHT OF THE BALL AND THE AREA ON THE COURT FROM WHICH IT WILL BE PLAYED. This concept and the rules (see rules section) require that players be aware of the flight of the ball and know where it will be played so that appropriate position adjustments can be made. The concepts of court positioning and how appropriate positioning is achieved must be taught.

It is necessary to teach racquetball skills with this strategical concept in mind and set performance goals so the players: a) can direct the ball to the area(s) on the court that are advantageous, b) use the strategy that provides for safe positioning in center court, and c) move and take a position in the correct relationship to the ball flight and the point at which it will be played by the opponent.

When in correct relationship to the hitter, it is appropriate for a player to "peek" over one shoulder to watch the opponent hit the ball. This is done by keeping the body facing forward, slightly turned toward the side of the court on which the ball will be played and turning the head to look over the shoulder. The player should **not turn and face the hitter.** A player should not be instructed to hit the ball and then back up into the center-court area no matter where the ball has gone. Neither should a player be instructed to simply crouch down if: 1) in the path of the ball as it travels to the front wall after being hit by the opponent, or 2) in the way of the opponent's swing. This is poor technique and should be corrected. INDIVIDUALS WHO PLAY THIS WAY SHOULD BE WARNED OF THE POTENTIAL DANGER IN THIS KIND OF PLAY AND INSTRUCTED IN APPROPRIATE COURT POSITIONING.

Drills used to teach court positioning can be developed by combining sequential returns of a single kind of shot between two players, i.e., backhand ceiling ball, or combination of shots, i.e., serve to the opponent's backhand, return of serve. An example of the first kind of drill would be:

> Player A sets a ceiling ball to player B's backhand and moves to the center court position in correct relationship to where the ball is on the court. Player B returns the ball with a ceiling ball to player A's backhand, forcing player A to move back and to

the backhand side while player B moves to the front court position.

Drills used to develop ball control and shot placement should be progressive from simple development of individual hitting techniques into a game-like setting. An example of this concept of progression would be: drop or toss the ball to self and hit, set the ball to self off the front wall and hit, take a set off the front wall from another player which requires moving to hit the ball, play the ball in a limited rally setting with another player focusing on a specific stroke and/or return area, then play in a game setting. Drills can be varied so that performers can practice under different conditions, considering the pace of the ball, position on the court, direction of the ball, etc. When designing drills it is important to remember that skills should always be practiced with a specific shot-target or shot-selection in mind—NEVER with the idea of simply hitting the ball "hard somewhere." Another example of a ball control and shot placement drill would be:

> Player A serves to player B on the backhand side and moves to the forecourt position. Player B returns the ball down to backhand side forcing player A to move deep and to the backhand while player B moves to the forecourt and takes correct position.

These are two simple examples of a great variety of drills that can be composed depending upon the skill level of the players, the skills being utilized, and the court circumstances being practiced.

While drills for court positioning and drills for ball control and placement have been discussed separately for the sake of emphasis and clarity, work on both aspects of play can be incorporated into individual drills.

Progression of Skills

The development of skills should, again, be in keeping with the concept of the game structure. Initially, students need to be able to hit a forehand pass, a forehand kill, a backhand pass, a backhand kill both down the wall and cross court, and a ceiling ball on both the forehand and backhand sides. Students also need to know serving skills, possibly the drive and lob serve, to both the opponent's forehand and backhand sides. Other skills which need to be included are: playing the ball off the backwall, positioning oneself in relation to where the ball will be played after rebounding from a side wall or more than one wall, and moving around another player or players.

In the development of skills, *emphasis should be on developing hitting technique and placement of shots, moving on the court* and *appropriately posi-*

tioning in relation to the hitter and the ball. More advanced shots or a greater variety of shots should not be attempted until the above basics have been mastered.

Physical Requirements of the Activity

There are no specific strength, flexibility, cardiorespiratory, or other conditioning requirements which are needed to offset the possibility of specific catastrophic injury. However, the higher the level of conditioning and preparation for participation, the less chance there will be that "accidents" will happen because of poor play habits or tiredness. There is a real danger that fatigue will cause a player to restrict movement, crowding another player when that player is hitting or not moving out of the way to allow the hitting player a clear shot to the front wall. From this perspective, fatigue can be a significant injury factor.

SPECIAL SAFETY CONSIDERATIONS

Rules of Play

The rules of play are written to encourage proper court positioning, thus reducing the chance of injury. A "hinder" may be called by the hitting player when the non-hitting player prohibits the hitting player from freely making the shot to which he or she is entitled.

Specific conditions that result in hinders include: 1) taking a position in line with the direct flight of the ball to the front wall; 2) not allowing the hitting player sufficient room to take a backswing without striking the non-hitting player; and 3) not allowing the hitting player sufficient room to play the ball.

Since hinders are called on the non-hitting player, the responsibility of the interference rests with that player. It does not matter whether the cause was: 1) lack of knowledge and ability to play appropriate positioning or 2) purposeful positioning to offset an advantage to the hitting player. The result is still a hinder.

In tournament settings an official calls hinders, and hinders result in loss of point or serve. (In games between high-level performers few hinders occur because of the ability to make appropriate shots and maintain court positioning.) In recreational or unofficiated games, it is difficult to call "hinders" and make service or point awards. In these situations the call of hinders usually results in the replay of the point since calls must be made by the players. The significant point is that the number of "hinder" situations, whether avoidable or not, is a clear barometer of the relative safety of the participants. Safety dictates that when there is no official, a hitting player should call "hinder" and replay the point rather than hit the other player with the ball or racquet. Some circumstances of play prohibit the hitting player from knowing where the non-hitting player is positioned, and one must rely on the non-hitting player to make appropriate court position adjustments to continue the play and avoid injury. If the non-hitting player does not watch the ball and take correct positioning action, the resulting situation can be extremely dangerous.

Often players are struck on the hitting player's follow-through. The rules indicate that this is not the fault of the hitting player, and a hinder will not be called unless the hitting player misses the intended shot as a result of the interference. Injuries resulting from being struck on the follow-through are usually more serious than those resulting from being struck on the backswing. This is because the racquet has travelled a greater distance and the individual is being struck with greater force.

Safety Equipment

Players should wear eye guards to protect the eyes from injury. Being struck by the ball in the eye or by a racquet in the temple or face can do severe damage. While lens-less eye guards provide some measure of safety, there have been instances where a direct hit by a ball has resulted in eye injury. Compression of the ball upon contact with the eye guard allows part of the ball to move into the open space of the eye guard and into the eye. The best eye protection requires guards which neither allow the ball to contact the eye because of compression on contact with the frames nor shatter when struck by a ball or racquet. This requires a lens style eyeguard and sturdy frames. The lenses should be polycarbonate plastic and frames polycarbonate injection-molded units. ASTM standard specifications should be used as the measure for eye protection devices. NO FEWER SAFETY PRECAUTIONS SHOULD BE TAKEN DURING PLAY BECAUSE PLAYERS HAVE EYE GUARDS.

The racquet must be attached to the player's wrist by a thong or string. Perspiration may cause the hand to become slippery and the thong insures that even though the grip may be lost, the racquet will not fly away from the player and cause injury.

Game of Doubles

The game of doubles is potentially more dangerous than singles. Since there are four players in the court, it is more difficult for players to avoid being in each other's way. Court positioning should be stressed, and *all* players need to be aware of the position of the ball at all times. In addition, players should be aware of possible "hinder" situations and the increased possibility of other players being hit with the ball and/or racquet. Players should be aware of and have an opportunity to practice basic doubles strategy, court positioning requirements, and individual responsibilities for court coverage under controlled conditions before being allowed to play under unsupervised conditions.

Instructor Supervision

Instruction in racquetball should include close supervision of all practice settings. The instructor should intervene to request the use of eye guards, or a more effective application of the calling of "hinders," or to assist players in developing a process of play which is safe and in keeping with the concept of the game.

This means that the instructor must have a functional understanding of the game, the shots, the rules, and the concept that effective play is also safe play. It must be understood and explained clearly to players, however, that because of the physical construction of racquetball/handball courts, it is impossible for an instructor to supervise safety in all courts simultaneously, and that all players acknowledge some responsibility for their own actions and safety in the court.

25

Squash Rackets

JANET K. DRAYDON
Polytechnic of North London
London, England

The game of squash rackets began at Harrow School in England in the mid-19th century, as the boys amused themselves in the courtyard while waiting to play racquets. It quickly spread to other schools in the private system and, importantly for its worldwide progress, into the British Army. Courts were built for Army officers at their postings in the British Empire, thus taking it to many countries. Many courts were built on the Indian sub-continent with the result that Pakistan now boasts many great male players. In the late 19th century the game arrived in the United States and Canada, and the first recorded individual championship in any country was held in the U.S. in 1906.

Today there are two forms of the game. Most of the squash-playing countries, and some clubs in the U.S., play the international game, whereas many clubs in the U.S. only play the American game. The international game has expanded in the U.S. somewhat of late due to the fact that Americans wish to compete on the international scene on equal terms with the rest of the squash-playing world. The main differences between the two games are: 1) the scoring system, 2) the dimensions of the court, and 3) the size and weight of the racket and ball.

However, both games have in common some potentially dangerous features. They are both played at high speed by two, or occasionally four, players jockeying for position in an enclosed area. Thus physical contact, body to body, or more dangerously, racket to body, is not only possible, but highly likely. A squash ball, in either version of the game, is small and, hard, and when hit very hard, can travel at speeds of up to 120 mph (Scrivener 1973). These two factors are the cause of most catastrophic injuries in squash (Table 25-1). It is the purpose of this chapter to suggest that many of these injuries could either be avoided altogether, or lessened in severity.

Table 25-1. Possible Catastrophic Injuries in Squash

Activity	Possible Injury	Cause	Prevention
Playing in spectacles/hard contact lenses, Player hit by ball or racket	Severe eye injury or loss of eye, Severe laceration to the face	Ball or racket hits eye, Spectacles shatter or hard contact lens lacerates eye	Spectacles should conform to safety specifications. Contact lenses should be soft
Player hit on head by ball or racket	Same as above	Ball or racket hits eye (often, but not always, caused by inadequate technique or control)	Adequate eye protection. Correct technique and knowledge of the rules
Player falls during play	Concussion	Player hits head against wall, Slippery floor surface, Incorrect footwear, Articles left on court floor	Maintenance of the floor surface, roof, and walls. Correct footwear
Strenuous play	Death	Coronory heart disease	Medical advice on health status. Sensible attitude to play if feeling ill. No total protection, but sensible precautions should minimize risk

POSSIBLE CATASTROPHIC INJURIES

Most catastrophic injuries occurring in squash are either to the eyes, or to the face and head area. Catastrophic injuries which have occurred are: 1) loss of, or more frequently, damage to vision, 2) severe lacerations to the face, 3) concussion, 4) broken limbs, and 5) death. Squash does not have a high rate of catastrophic injuries, and certainly does not have a high death rate. Yet several cases of 'sudden death' on the squash court have been documented in recent years, in both world class and recreational competition. In all cases these have been due to heart failure during or following exertion on the squash court.

FACTORS CAUSING CATASTROPHIC INJURIES

Injuries to the eye and face are by far the most common and are caused by the following situations:
1. The ball is driven at speed into the player's eye.
2. The ball shatters the player's spectacles.

3. The player is hit in the eye or face by the opponent's racket during backswing or follow-through.
4. The player's spectacles are shattered by the opponent's racket during backswing or follow-through.

These injuries are usually the result of faulty technique on the part of one or both players, and are not only found in novice play.

Other injuries have been caused by the following situations:
5. The player falls, crashing into the sidewall of the court.
6. The player crashes into the handle of the door in the backwall of the court, the handle being left in the open position.
7. The player has an existing cardiac condition.
8. The ball gets caught in the lights, or on a ledge surrounding the court, and the player falls while trying to retrieve it.

INSTRUCTOR RESPONSIBILITY IN PREVENTING CATASTROPHIC INJURIES

Squash is an exciting, fast-moving game. Yet to see an expert squash game in slow motion is almost like witnessing an intricately choreographed dance scene as the players weave and glide past each other, touching or almost touching much of the time. Since the squash ball travels at speeds of up to 120 mph, and fits neatly into the orbital cavity of the eye, the potential for harm is great. Yet injuries are not common, and have been estimated at between 1.7 and 9.4 injuries per 100,000 games (Scrivener 1973). Students should be told of this but warned that injuries, when they occur, can be severe. It is the responsibility of both instructor and players to ensure that safety precautions are understood and practiced.

Because the types of injuries which occur in squash tend to fall into distinct categories, the following discussion will take each in turn.

INJURIES TO THE EYES AND FACE FROM BALL AND RACKET

It has been shown (Barrell et al. 1981; Clemett and Fairhurst 1980; Easterbrook 1982; Ingram 1973) that most catastrophic injuries in squash are to the eyes, and are caused by squash balls being driven at the eye at great speeds. Both the North American ball and the international ball fit extremely well into the orbit of the eye. It is for this reason that eye injuries, when they occur, can be very serious. Estimates of the rates of injury vary between 3.7 (Barrell et al. 1981) and 9.4 (Clemett and Fairhurst 1980) per 100,000 competitive sessions played. Clearly these rates are not excessively high, yet damage may be severe, causing some permanent reduction in visual acuity in many instances, blindness, or the removal of the damaged eye.

Players who seem to be most at risk of suffering permanent damage are spectacle and contact lens wearers, particularly myopes. If spectacle lenses are smashed, glass or plastic often enters the eye, causing extensive damage. It is important to note that hardened glass spectacle lenses do not protect from injury, as they too will often shatter when hit by the squash ball or racket. Plastic lenses too may shatter if not of adequate thickness. There are several eye protectors currently on the market, aiming to prevent eye damage. Unfortunately, many of them do not offer adequate protection. It has been found (Easterbrook 1982) that those consisting merely of frames without any plastic lenses inside them, serve only to compress the ball and funnel it into the eye.

As well as catastrophic injuries caused by the ball, there are many injuries to the eyes and face caused by the opponent's racket, exacerbated in some instances by spectacle lenses breaking, or by metal spectacle frames lacerating the bridge of the nose.

Catastrophic injuries are not only the prerogative of the novice player. They can occur in players of many years experience, yet there are often faults of technique which contribute significantly to eye and face injuries.

There are several safety points that the instructor and player should be aware of, some of them relating to eye wear, the others relating to technique:

1. If the player wears spectacles, the lenses should be made of polycarbonate or industrial safety 3 millimeter center thickness CR39 plastic, never of glass, whether hardened or not. It has been found that ordinary street-wear glasses, even with lenses made of plastic, do not afford adequate protection (Easterbrook 1982). The thickness of the plastic lens at its minimum point should be no less than 3 millimeters. Refer to the standard described in the racquetball chapter.
2. Spectacle frames should be of nylon with rubber padding at the bridge of the nose.
3. Player who wear contact lenses should be counselled to wear the soft type.
4. Eye guards, with plastic or polycarbonate lenses, either plain or prescription, are recommended by many medical practitioners. The instrutor should outline the dangers to contact lens wearers, particularly those wearing hard lenses, and counsel them about eyeguards. It has been estimated that only about 1.4 percent of players actually do wear eyeguards, despite the dangers (Clemett and Fairhurst 1980). Many players feel the eyeguards are uncomfortable and hamper their game. That is a decision that only the player can make—the instructor's task is to outline the options available to players.

5. Rackets must be kept in good repair. A racket which has been damaged so that it has become a potential hazard should not be used for play, If repaired, the material should have a smooth surface. The grip should not be allowed to become smooth and slippery, or it may fly out of the player's hand during the execution of a stroke. Worn grips, either towelling or leather, should be replaced. It is possible to use a thong which is attached to the racket handle and which fits around the player's wrist to prevent this danger. Some players prefer to wear a leather glove on the racket hand.

6. Players should be taught correct striking technique. The wrist should be cocked, and the elbow bent on the backswing; the follow through should be upwards, not around the body, and should be controlled at all times.

7. Players should be taught not to crowd their opponents, particularly on the opponent's backhand side of the court, as the backhand follow-through is typically wider than the forehand for most players. Many racket injuries are caused in this way.

8. Players should be instructed to watch the ball as far as possible onto the opponent's racket, turning to watch the ball into the back of the court. A common fault with novice players is that they stare intently at the front wall waiting for the ball to come from behind them. It is precisely then that if they turn, wondering what has happened to the ball, they can be hit in the eye. Only by watching the ball into the back of the court can the player know where the ball is, and be aware of what the opponent is aiming to do.

9. Instructors should discourage the technique of "turning." This consists of following the ball into one of the corners, usually the backhand corner, letting it go round the corner and out onto the player's other side (Figure 25-1), then turning and hitting, usually at full power, a stroke down the middle of the court. The player thus plays a forehand on the backhand side of the court and vice versa. It has been argued that a player can only turn off a bad length shot, thus it is the opponent's fault for playing badly and encouraging turning. While this is undoubtedly true, it remains the case that turning, while perfectly legal, is extremely dangerous and to be discouraged.

10. Novices should learn to play a controlled game of singles before they are introduced to doubles. Four people on a squash court are a crowd, only players in control of themselves and their games should be encouraged to play with partners.

11. Instructors should ensure that players are familiar with the rules relating to 'let ball' and 'stroke.' Many accidents could be pre-

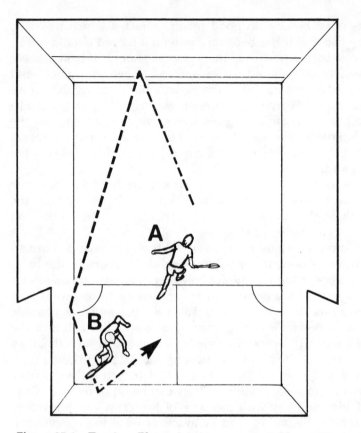

Figure 25-1. Turning. Player A is in a very turnable position as Player B "turns" off a bad length shot.

vented if players would ask for a 'let' (also referred to as a 'hinder') when they feel their opponent is obstructing their free strike at the ball.

12. Players should wear white or pastel colored squash clothing, as dark clothing is a poor backcloth against which to see a dark squash ball. It is essential to be able to see the ball at all times.

SUDDEN DEATH

Sudden death is normally defined as death occurring one to 24 hours after the onset of symptoms (Northcote, Evans, and Ballantine 1984). A report of sudden death in squash players has shown that death commonly occurs within six hours of playing, with most documented cases occurring actually on the court. Most of these players had complained recently of a change in perceived health status, many had documented cardiovascular irregularities, yet they continued to play squash.

It is tempting to suggest that players, particularly those of middle-age who have been otherwise sedentary, should have a medical check-up before starting to play squash. Yet many athletes show 'positive tests,' and many 'negative tests' have been reported on runners who subsequently suffer sudden death (Tunstall 1984). Thus, it is difficult to be prescriptive. Squash players may be particularly prone to sudden death, but in most cases there are existing, if undiagnosed, cardiovascular abnormalities. It is likely that these players would have died prematurely anyway. Squash may have precipitated the death in the way that taking an elderly car on a long freeway drive may cause its premature demise.

However, the instructor and player each have their responsibilities:
1. The instructor who wishes to teach middle-aged and older players should be familiar with the signs of cardiorespiratory distress, and optimally, be familiar with resuscitative techniques.
2. The instructor should ensure that players, particularly those taking up the game in middle age, report any adverse symptoms to their medical practitioners.
3. Players should be discouraged from playing if they feel ill, however temporary they imagine the symptoms to be.
4. Middle-aged and older players should step up the intensity and duration of their exercise gradually.

It is also worth noting that sudden death in squash seems to be a mainly masculine event. The reasons for this remain unclear. It may be due to the higher incidence of coronary heart disease in males, or due to the fact that more males than females play the game, or that males play more intensely, or a combination of these factors.

CONCUSSION/BROKEN LIMBS/OTHER

Concussion in squash is normally the result of the player slipping and crashing the head against the extremely hard sidewall. It is not a common event, and when it occurs is usually the result of an inadequate floor surface and/or inappropriate footwear. It can also occur if the player is hit on the head by the opponent's racket.

Broken limbs are also extremely rare, but have they been known to occur when a player attempts to retrieve a ball from the lights above the court or from a ledge around the court.

The instructor should ensure therefore that:
1. The floor has not become slippery through prolonged use; it must be resanded regularly.
2. There is no moisture on the court, either from a leaky roof or

walls, from 'sweating' courts, or from excessive perspiration from previous users.

3. Footwear should be light and flexible, yet should grip the court easily but not rigidly. Squash shoes should have ridged soles; they should not be smooth through use. It is false economy to use a pair of old shoes that have "lost their grip" on the court. Squash shoes should not be worn outdoors, they should be kept for the squash court or gymnasium only.

4. Ideally the court should have two small covered recesses in the 'tin' section of the front wall for players' valuables. If there are none and valuables must be taken on the court for security reasons, they should be placed in the front corners, never the back corners where a player may slip on them.

5. Players should never be allowed to climb around the court to retrieve the ball, however tempting it may appear. This may sound rather extreme, but broken limbs have been caused by this foolhardy behavior.

Other safety factors concern the door which normally opens directly from the backwall into the squash court. It normally has a metal handle, which, when opened to exit from the court, protrudes into the court. It can cause injuries, and should be in the flush position when play is in progress. Injuries can also occur if the door is unexpectedly opened during play. Waiting players should not open the door unless they have ascertained that there is no one on the court.

6. Players should close the handle of the door, which is usually in the backwall, so that it is flush with the wall. Some injuries are caused by players hitting their heads on an open handle.

7. The instructor should never allow players to enter the squash court where play is, or may be, in progress, without first knocking and waiting for the occupants to open the door.

SKILL DEVELOPMENT

It has been estimated that the squash racket can travel at speeds of up to 125 m.p.h. One of the most important, if not the most important safety factor, is that the player must be in control of the racket at all times. Wild hitting is to be discouraged at every opportunity. It is not good squash, it does not promote skill development, and it is highly dangerous.

Novice players should be taught that control is essential at all times for player safety. For the instructor teaching a group of novices, practices should emphasize control and accuracy:

1. Students should learn to hit a straight ball down the sidewall. The instructor should demonstrate correct technique which emphasizes a swing restricted in its diameter by elbow flexion and

the 'cocking' of the wrist. Players coming to the game from tennis are particularly prone to exhibit an incorrect and wide swing. It is the responsibility of the instructor to correct a wide swing, not only for reasons of safety, but because it will inhibit correct technique for extracting the ball from the back corners of the court. Lack of skill in this area will always restrict a player's progress in the game.

2. Students should be taught to keep the ball away from the center of the court. A ball hit down the middle of the court is always a potential hazard as both players jockey for position in the area of the "T."

3. Students should be introduced to the rules governing 'let ball' and 'stroke' as soon as they attempt any competitive play. Briefly, these rules state that a player must have a fair view of the ball and must be free to hit the ball to any area of the front wall. It is difficult to overemphasize the importance of a knowledge of these rules, as many injuries would be prevented if only players would realize that they are entitled to ask for a 'let' (and possibly get a 'stroke') if they feel their shot is being hampered by the presence of their opponent, or if they feel that by hitting the ball they will 'drill' it at the opponent.

4. Students should be taught that they should always watch the ball into the back of the court when their opponent is behind them.

5. When, and only when, the instructor can set up a safe situation should the student be encouraged to let go and hit the ball as hard as possible. It is very satisfying to hit the ball hard, to hear the crack it makes on the front wall, and students should experience this pleasure. However, in the interests of skill as well as safety it has to be planned.

6. Students should be taught the value of a "good length ball", i.e., a ball which, on its second bounce arrives at the back wall, preferably in one of the corners. Such technique will discourage the dangerous practice of "turning," as it is impossible to turn off a good length ball, either straight or cross court.

SPECIAL SAFETY CONSIDERATIONS

Equipment

Students should be made aware of the dangers of eye injury and alerted to the possible precautions outlined previously. Footwear should be kept especially for the squash court, and should not be allowed to wear until slippery. Damaged rackets should be either replaced or properly repaired. Handle grips should be replaced if they have become smooth.

Facilities

It is recommended that the floor be made of Canadian maple or beech, for reasons of hardness and color. It should be resurfaced regularly to prevent it becoming smooth and shiny. Any broken or uneven floorboards should be mended or replaced. The roof and walls of the court must kept in good repair so that moisture from rain or condensation is not allowed to collect on the court.

Technique

Players should learn correct technique from the very beginning. They should also learn that squash is not a game of wild hitting, it is a game of control.

Officials

Competitive play should be controlled by competent markers and referees who will not hesitate to make firm decisions in the case of dangerous play, to the point of disqualifying a player who persists in playing dangerously when warned. Players should have confidence that they will be awarded a let or stroke if they hold shots because of the danger of hitting opponents with either rackets or balls.

26

Tennis

REX DAVIS
Washington State University
Pullman, Washington

While the number of possible catastrophic injuries attributed to tennis is minimal, there are situations for concern (Table 26-1). These situations need to be discussed with the players prior to the season so that they will be aware of their importance. The means for prevention should also be discussed and consciously included in the teaching of techniques and knowledge of players.

POSSIBLE CATASTROPHIC INJURIES IN TENNIS

Catastrophic injuries in tennis include:
1. Heatstroke resulting from extended play under very warm, sunny, humid conditions.
2. A ball striking a player in the eye as the result of a hit by another player, usually a partner or opponent in doubles. Eye protective devices as indicated for racquetball may be recommended for tennis. Net position play and overhead volleys from the opponent are situations in which players may not be able to respond quickly enough to prevent the ball from striking the eye. Therefore, players should be informed that eye protection devices are available.
3. Severe head injury from running into a net post, falling, or tripping when attempting to jump the net.
4. Severe neck and head injuries resulting from running into the fence at the back or sides of the court.

PREVENTION OF CATASTROPHIC INJURY

Players should be given warnings of dangers and dangerous behaviors. In particular they should be warned of the following catastrophic injury-producing situations:

Table 26-1. Possible Catastrophic Injuries in Tennis

Activity	Possible Injury	Cause	Prevention
Jumping the net	Head injury, Brain damage	Catching a foot or lower leg, Falling forward on head	Don't jump the net
Running into net post or fence	Head injury, Neck injury	Attempting to retrieve ball beyond reach, Running into obstruction	Player alertness. Knowledge of the court and obstructions
Playing in extremely hot or humid climate	Heatstroke	Overheating, Lack of perspiration, Inadequate water intake, Dehydration	Conditioning in hot temperatures. Maintaining an adequate water intake. Wearing a cap or head covering
Rally in doubles	Loss of sight in eye	Direct hit to eye	Player alertness. Reaction drills as a regular part of practice. Wear eye protection devices

1. A. During hot weather, particularly on sunny and humid days, heat stroke is a possibility. Water intake should be maintained during a match or practice to avoid dehydration.
   B. If a player's skin becomes hot and dry, and there is no perspiration, immediate action should be taken by applying ice or cold towels and seeking of medical attention.
2. Eye injury can result from being hit in the eyeball with the ball. Hitting a ball at an unsuspecting player "for fun" or just giving it a hit out of frustration when the ball is not in play can result in serious injury. When playing doubles, players should be alert for any shot which might be hit towards them, even if they do not seem to be involved in the point.
3. Tennis courts vary in the distance provided between the court boundaries and the back fence or side fence. Not being aware of these distances puts a player in a possible injury situation.
4. Jumping the net is not wise and should not be attempted. Catching a foot or feet results in a headlong fall with little chance of protecting oneself from possible severe head, face, or neck injury.

Correct Technique to Avoid Injury

The cause of catastrophic injury in tennis is not usually the technique used to strike the ball. As can be seen from the kinds of injuries listed and the warnings, the usual causes are careless play or lack of awareness of playing circumstances.

Knowledgeable and alert play during doubles should be taught, not only to increase the opportunity for winning, but also to avoid injury. The frequency of hits, particularly during close net play, requires that all players be "into the point" and be alert that a ball might suddenly be hit at them. A slow reaction could lead to an eye injury.

Practice drills should be utilized in which court dimensions, obstacles, and locomotor patterns are synthesized and "memorized."

Physical Requirements of the Activity

Although a person who is well conditioned may still succumb to heat stroke if the body's fluid level drops or if he or she remains in the sun too long, a good conditioning program can contribute to prevention of such difficulties. In addition, coaches should teach players to take small amounts of water during a match or practice when body fluid is being lost.

There are no specific conditioning requirements that will guarantee that no catastrophic injury can occur. However, the better the condition of the player, the less likely that fatigue will result in some unforeseen "accident."

SPECIAL SAFETY CONSIDERATIONS

Overall, tennis is a relatively safe game with regard to catastrophic injuries. As in other "safe" circumstances it is usually some careless act which results in an injury. Therefore, a coach should discourage such behaviors as throwing a racquet, carelessly hitting a ball to someone who isn't looking, or taking the frustration of a poor hit or bad play by hitting the ball toward or across the net with great force.

27

Track and Field

ROBERT CASSLEMAN
Washington State University
Pullman, Washington

Track and field is a sport which can be both the safest and most dangerous of organized sports on the grade school, high school, and college levels. The 20 individual and team events have different characteristics and are performed at different sites. Thus it is mandatory that the coach/teacher/organizer be familiar with all the events and be aware of potential risks in each (Table 27-1). The determining factors in the safe execution of each event include the proper use of well-maintained equipment, knowledge of correct techniques by coaches and athletes, appropriate supervision, and properly organized practices and competition.

The 20 different events in track and field should be divided into three main areas: throwing, jumping, and running. Each area involves different kinds and degrees of risk, and only a few of the total number of events are of major concern with respect to catastrophic injury. Throwing events involve the propulsion of an implement into the air; jumping events involve an airborne phase of the athlete; and running events can require that a large proportion of training be done away from the direct supervision of the coach, for example, distance running.

POSSIBLE CATASTROPHIC INJURIES

Most accidental catastrophic injuries that occur during participation in the throwing events include injuries involving impact of airborne projectiles: concussion, skull fracturing, and stabbing wounds. The distance covered by the implements, their speed, and the unpredictability of their landing are the main reasons why throwing events are dangerous. In the hammer throw, the maintenance of the implement is of major concern. The lack of awareness of the environment on the part of participants and spectators, combined with the fact that in track and field

Table 27-1. Possible Catastrophic Injuries in Track and Field

Activity	Possible Injury	Cause	Prevention
Javelin throw	Trauma to major organs (circulatory to nervous pathway), Death, Puncture wounds	Impact of the javelin	Instruct athletes not to throw when non-participants are wandering around throwing area. Clearly mark or restrict throwing/landing area with pennants, rope, or fencing. Place practice area away from track and infield, especially during learning stage, and when there are different groups of athletes on the field. Control traffic inside the landing sector during a meet. Designate a Marshall. When teaching the students how to throw, have all the athletes throw before retrieving the javelins. Throwers should wait until coach signals before retrieving implements
Hammer and discus throws, Shot put	Trauma to major organs, Concussion, Damage to the spinal cord and head, Broken neck, Skull fracture	Impact of a projectile	Have a cage enclosing at least ¾ of the circle. Instruct other athletes to be aware of throwing dangers. Keep the implement in good condition (check wires and handles in the hammer). Do not allow throwing when facilities are inadequate (no cage, not enough space). Warn all persons within the possible range of the path of an airborne implement (members of the coaching staff, managers) of the danger involved. All persons not directly involved with the track and field team should be prohibited entirely from throwing event areas. At competitive sites, access to the throwing sectors should be restricted to event officials, coaches, and event participants. Participants should be taught to look before throwing. Encourage throwers to work with each other, or under a coach's supervision at all times

Table 27-1. Possible Catastrophic Injuries in Track and Field *(Continued)*

Distance running	Struck by a motor vehicle	The possible catastrophic injuries to a distance runner would number any one of the many injuries that could be sustained by a pedestrian (injury by impact of an automobile, or other moving object). Injuries could be to the head or spinal column, and could include death	Coaches should instruct runners to run facing the opposite direction of the traffic flow when running on the roads. Avoid heavily traveled roads or busy streets. Cross roads only at pedestrian crosswalks or intersections. Runners should follow pedestrian rules. Avoid thoroughfares that do not have sidewalks. Run on shoulder of road, not pavement, when there is no sidewalk available. Avoid areas where farming equipment is being used. Run single file. Front and back runners should make other athletes aware of possible dangers. Warn of oncoming traffic
	Impairment of thermoregulatory system	Heat stroke	Administration of sufficient liquids before, during, and after workouts. Avoid running during peak temperature hours and high levels of humidity. Acclimate runners to hot temperatures through use of progressively longer exposures to heat
Hurdling	Hurdler hits hurdle placed in opposite direction. Catching the hurdle with leg or foot	Broken neck, Concussion	Teach proper hurdling technique. Teach proper use of hurdle (hurdles are built to fall in one direction—built to be knocked over in one direction)
Vertical jumps: pole vault	Missing the pit on landing, Inadequate landing pit	Concussion, Death, Injury to back and neck soft tissue, Fractures to back and neck	Landing pit meets guidelines in National Federation of High School (NFHS) or International Amateur Athletics Federation (IAAF) guidebooks. Cover base of crossbar standards with six inches of foam padding. Have person stationed near

(continued)

Table 27-1. Possible Catastrophic Injuries in Track and Field (*Continued*)

Activity	Possible Injury	Cause	Prevention
			plant box to catch vaulting pole before it strikes ground or standards. Match vaulting pole size to individual vaulter's characteristics. Avoid poles that are too light in weight. Maintain speed throughout entire run up. Do not practice when extremely tired
Vertical jumps: high jump	Concussion, Death, Injury to back and neck soft tissue, Fractures to back and neck	Missing the pit on landing, Inadequate landing pit	Teaching proper landing technique. Landing pit meets guidelines in NFHS, National Collegiate Athletic Association (NCAA), or IAAF. Have adequate equipment. Maintain it in good condition. Teach events in a reasonable progression and proper landing technique (upper body, head tucked). Landing area should be soft and of adequate size. (Check on possible holes caused by overuse.) Always work out under supervision of a coach. Do not practice when extremely tired

a number of events are taking place at one time, generates risk. Athletes, coaches, officials, and on occasions spectators, become so involved in their own activities that they lose perception of the potential danger from other activities. Very often, people cross throwing sectors without realizing what they are doing.

Vertical jumping events include an airborne phase and a landing phase which can place vital body parts in a position vulnerable to injury at impact. The major risks in these events involve landing on the head, which can cause severe damage to the nervous system, the spinal cord, and/or the neck due to a technical error in the execution of the event. Inappropriate, insufficient, and poorly maintained equipment (combined with erroneous technique) is also a common cause of catastrophic injuries (e.g., landing pit not large enough, resulting in the athlete missing the landing pit completely, or the vaulting pole breaking because it is not stiff enough).

Possible catastrophic injuries to runners, although uncommon, need to be brought to the attention of participants. Those injuries would number any one of the many injuries that could be sustained by a pedestrian (injured by the impact of a moving vehicle). Injuries could be anything from a concussion, to spinal cord damage, to death. The unawareness of possible dangers while running on the roads and the assumption that all drivers will be aware of a runner and will be able to stop for them is the major cause of accidents among runners. Within the running events, hurdling should be mentioned as a potential risk for a broken neck and concussion. Although not common as a major cause of catastrophic injuries, hurdling could be dangerous if an athlete runs over a hurdle placed in the wrong direction, or uses an improper technique causing him/her to flip over the hurdle and land on the back, neck, or head.

PREVENTION OF CATASTROPHIC INJURIES

As a general rule, prior to participation in any activity in track and field, coaches and administrators have to require physical examinations for all prospective student-athletes. As practices start, but before coaching or instruction begins each season, it is the best interest of the coach to warn all candidates that the activities they are involved in have the risk of catastrophic injury

Throwing

Throwers should be advised that attentiveness to instruction, awareness of activities around the throwing area, responsibility for throwing and retrieving, and having the proper and well maintained equipment are the major ways to avoid injuries. Landing sectors should be of limited access and they should be roped off to ensure safety of other track athletes, spectators, and coaches. During instruction periods, throwers have to be advised not to throw until the instructor or coach allows them to do so, and not to retrieve implements until all the throwers have completed their throws.

Within the category of throwing events, there are safety considerations for each event. In the shot put, the main concern should simply be the awareness that the implement is being thrown. The flight of the shot is shorter and is more predictable than other throws, but individuals who are not involved in the event frequently cross through the landing area without realizing the potential danger. While an athlete is throwing, other throwers and coaches should be aware of any person attempting to cross in front of the throw, since the shot putter starts the movements facing the opposite direction to the landing area. In the past few years the rotational technique in the shot put has gained some popularity, adding extra concerns in terms of safety. While in the O'Brien (traditional) technique, the shot describes a linear path, in the rotational technique a circular path is described by the shot while the athlete completes the turns in the circle, generating centrifugal forces. Keeping control of the shot while turning one and a half times until a controlled release is achieved is of the greatest concern to athletes and coaches. The shot has to be kept in contact with the neck until the moment of the release. This is a rule which should be enforced to avoid uncontrolled releases.

Discus and hammer throwers incur similar risks as shot putters using rotational technique, but to a larger scale. Throwers have less control over the implement while generating speed and force as they complete their turns in the circle. To provide some protection to athletes, coaches, and spectators, all hammer throws should be made from a cage built around the circle. The same cage could be used for the discus.

If there is no cage available for the discus, coaches, and athletes should be advised to stand behind and away from the circle, or in the opposite side to the circle from where the discus will be released (left side of circle - when facing the direction of the throw - for right hand throwers).

In the hammer throw, athletes should be advised of the importance of checking the implement before each throw. The handle, wire, and hammer head should be securely fastened such that they will not separate during the winds or turns.

The height, distance, and speed that the implements achieve in flight join together for unpredictable landings. The landing areas for these events are very extensive in size. This apparent "open space" becomes a temptation for others not involved in the event to cut across the sector. Also the fact that there is "dead time" between throws makes athletes, spectators, and coaches lose awareness that the event is taking place. Because of these factors, landing areas should be roped off. Participants should be taught to look before throwing, and another person (athlete, coach, official) should monitor the landing area.

Jumping

In track and field, adherence to proper technique to produce the ultimate in performance is likewise the best way to prevent injuries. The events in track and field in which proper execution of the correct technique is most crucial in avoiding injuries are the vertical jumps: high jump and pole vault.

High jump and pole vault are two very attractive events for newcomers in track and field. Certain fascination exists among young people who want to experience an airborne sensation and landing on a soft pit. Instructors and coaches have to make athletes aware of the potential danger of playing around the pit without the proper knowledge of the event.

The school or institution hosting workout sessions and competition for pole vaulting is responsible for providing safe facilities and proper equipment. Guidelines for landing pit dimensions are contained in the guidebook for the National Federation of High Schools (NFHS), National Collegiate Athletic Association (NCAA) and International Amateur Athletic Federation (IAAF). As an appendage to the above guidelines it is recommended that the base of the standards be covered with padding and that the pole vault landing pit extend toward the runway to border both sides of the plant box. The landing pits should be made of a composition which will allow a comfortable landing. For the high jump the pit should be a minimum height of 70 centimeters (28 inches), minimum dimensions of 4.88 by 2.44 meters (16 x 8 feet). A depth of 3.05 meters (10 feet) is recommended. The distance from the mat to the bar should not exceed 60 to 70 centimeters for beginners. The pole vault pit needs to be of a minimum of 4.88 meters wide by 3.66 meters deep (16 x 12 feet); beyond the vertical plane of the stop board a depth of 4.88 meters (16 feet) of landing surface is recommended. The material in the pit should be 91.44 centimeters (36 inches). ASTM current specifications for dimensions and impact/rebound characteristics should be checked.

High Jump Technique: Although the occurrence of catastrophic injury sustained in high jumping is rare, the potential does exist. The main area of concern is the landing position when using the Fosbury Flop technique. The approach, take-off, and bar clearance are of lesser importance, although lack of control in the approach and take-off may result in crashing into the standard. A catastrophic injury could occur if an athlete, in the landing phase, misses the landing pit completely and hits the back or head on the ground or incorrectly on the pit. Control in approach and take-off phases is important in order to have a controlled and appropriate landing. An appropriate and safe landing is one where the athlete lands contacting the pit with the upper back while the head is tucked.

For a safe landing in the high jump, the body assumes an L-position or pike after clearing the bar with the hips. This is achieved by tucking chin to the chest, lifting the legs, contracting the hip flexors. Experience for the landing action is gained through a variety of practices, especially falling and landing exercises.

The basic exercises for bar clearance and appropriate movements in mid-air and landing are:

1. Mobility drills mainly at hip level.
2. Acrobatics on mat, and agility exercises related to jumping.
3. Standing facing away from the pit with the bar slightly above hip level, the athlete takes off powerfully from both feet. The hips are extended and brought up and forward (arching) while legs are kept hanging loose. The arched position is maintained until the hips have cleared the bar. Then the hips are flexed, legs are lifted up, and the head is tucked achieving an L-position with the body. (The head is never thrown back while going over the bar. The head is turned towards the shoulder on the same side as the lead leg.)
4. Same exercise as above, but take off from a platform which allows a longer flight time.

The athlete has to be discouraged from landing with the neck or head as a point of contact, even on a soft landing pit.

Since the rotational movements are largely determined during the plant/take-off stage, it is very important for the coach to provide adequate supervision, evaluation, and feedback during the learning stages of the whole technique.

Pole Vault Technique: Injuries incurred while participating in pole vaulting include paraplegia, quadriplegia, and death resulting from damage to the spinal cord, caused by impact at landing of the vaulter's head, neck, or back on hard surfaces. These can include the exposed ground, the runway surface, the plant box, the crossbar support standard, or cement pads underneath the standards. The potential vaulter should be warned of the inherent risk of injury involved with participation prior to the first practice session.

Choosing the proper pole is important. The athlete's weight, the height at which the upper hand grips the pole, and the speed attained at take-off are the main factors in pole selection. The pole manufacturers give recommendations for matching pole to the athlete. Too light a pole can break resulting in injury from the pole or landing outside the dimensions of the pit. The coach should stress proper care of the pole to avoid cracks, dents, or other exterior damage.

Most errors in technique in the pole vault have their origin during the plant and take-off. According to Steve Miller, a coach for the Olympic Development Program for the pole vault, probably the single most dangerous technique error is a loss in approach speed in the last few strides. Beginning vaulters must learn to maintain running speed throughout the entire approach. In this way the vaulter is almost assured to land in the padded pit, regardless of subsequent mistakes in the attempt.

Vaulters must be told to abort any trials in which improper plant of pole, loss of control, excess veering to the right or left of the line of travel, or inadequate momentum exist. The vaulter must be made to realize that the landing pit is designed to protect landings of reasonably correct vaults and cannot protect in situations where vaults should not have been attempted. Particularly in a competitive situation, vaulters must be reminded to abort a trial when conditions are such that a catastrophic injury would probably occur should the athlete attempt "to save the vault."

Running

Although catastrophic injury as a result of running is rare, there are two situations that can result in serious injury: being struck by an automobile, and illness due to overexposure to heat. The types of traffic-related injuries sustained by runners are the same as those suffered by other pedestrians. To avoid liability problems, it is advisable for the coach to warn the runners prior to the season turnout that there is a risk of injury when training on the road. Of the countless circumstances that could be envisioned, the following suggestions should be given greatest emphasis:

1. When running along a road or its shoulder, run in the direction opposite the flow of traffic.
2. Wear bright or reflective clothing when running at any time, day or night.
3. When running in groups, run in a single file line.
4. Obey all traffic laws.

Catastrophic injuries can occur in runners as a result of illness from overexposure to heat. In cases where patients recover from heat stroke, irreversible damage to the nervous system can remain, including impairment of the thermoregulatory function of the hypothalamus.

From an instructional standpoint it is important to inform the runner that it is vitally important to drink water and other fluid replacements on a regular basis, especially during hot weather. Fluids should be consumed in the regular diet, during workouts, and before and during competition, when practical. It may be useful to mention that research has not shown water intake to be detrimental to running performance.

From a coaching standpoint it would be helpful to acclimatize or adapt the runners to unusually warm ambient temperatures to avoid the risk of heat disorders. This can be achieved with a progressive training schedule that exposes the team to longer bouts of exercise from day to day over a five-to eight-day period. The American College of Sports Medicine issued a position paper recommending measures to be taken by race organizers and athletes when participating in distance races (Mathews and Fox 1976). These recommendations have been incorporated into the preceding paragraphs.

28

Wrestling

LES HOGAN
Alaska Pacific University
Anchorage, Alaska

Because of the contact nature of the sport of wrestling, there are many potential situations for catastrophic injuries. The purpose of this chapter is to help the reader realize these situations, be aware of their causes, and understand the instructional responsibility of the coach.

One of the primary catastrophic injuries in wrestling is the fracture of the neck or back. Usually these types of injuries can be prevented by assuring that each wrestler completely understands the rules of the sport. It is imperative that the coach has knowledge of the skill levels and physiological ages of the athletes being coached. Ask the questions: "What can this group do safely?" and "What can't they do safely?"

It is imperative that the mat area and workout area are well padded and kept in repair. A coach must understand and use correct conditioning and weight training methods. Internal rupture, punctured internal organs, and concussions are usually the result of one or more of the above mentioned factors. Coaches must teach rules, know the human body, understand strength and conditioning techniques, and be aware of growth and development stages of young athletes.

A second area of potential danger is caused by lack of proper knowledge of weight control. Coaches should understand the human body and what happens if there is a change in water content, food intake, basal metabolism, or any drastic change to the system. Coaches must monitor each athlete to be alert to changes in weight. A coach should also be cognizant of changes in personality, school attendance, excessive nose bleeds, drop in grades, or lack of energy and strength.

A third area is in teaching technique. A coach must know the level of skill of each athlete so that skills are not taught beyond the knowledge or physical ability of the athlete. For example, it would be poor practice to teach upper body throws to a physically immature boy. Further, the coach should understand the potential dangers involved with each technique as well as what makes a move legal or illegal (e.g., a throw versus a forceful throw).

PROGRESSION OF SKILLS

Some guidelines for teaching progression include:

1. Assess the level of the athletes

A. Physically—strength and maturity
B. Skill—knowledge and ability to perform at the level being taught.

2. Perform a task analysis of each skill to be taught

For example, in order to teach a pinning combination, this is the order of knowledge: A. position, B. motion, C. breakdowns, D. rides, and E. pins.

3. Monitoring

It is imperative in skill development that learning is monitored. A new or advanced skill should not be introduced until the previous skill has been learned and mastered.

4. Adjusting

As skills are introduced, a coach usually discovers that certain athletes cannot learn certain skills. It might be caused by lack of mastery of an earlier skill, or it might be caused by a physical fact (e.g., body type, lack of balance). Therefore, a coach will have to adjust skills taught based upon individuals, not upon expectations. This doesn't mean individualizing the workout to a one-on-one. More than likely, groups of athletes can learn certain skills and other groups can learn another set of skills.

5. Basic Philosophy

Skills should be taught only if they fit into an overall coaching philosophy. The philosophy should fit into all situations that occur and should be easily understood by the athletes. It is impossible to teach a skill to cover every situation that occurs in wrestling. Therefore, a basic philosophy in coaching allows wrestlers an opportunity to adjust actions to a few basic rules. For example, at North Idaho College men's wrestling team, philosophy involves two skills, basic position and basic motion. At any time in any situation, if a wrestler is in poor position or if his motion stops before it should, he knows the action was incorrect and that he will have to adjust. This allows great flexibility in group teaching and it also allows the athlete to know instantly what needs to be changed in any situation.

CONDITIONING OF PARTICIPANTS

1. Training Programs

Training program will vary according to the personal philosophy of the coaches. There are, today, successful programs that mostly drill, those that mostly exercise, and those that mostly scrimmage. All are effective. However, all follow similar guidelines in practice sessions. These guidelines consider:
A. Skill level of athlete
B. Physical level of the athlete
C. BEFORE EACH PRACTICE answer the 3H's
   1. how much?
   2. how long?
   3. how often?
D. adjusting as the season progresses

2. Strength programs

Today, more than ever before, strength has become an integral part of wrestling. If some wrestlers are weak in comparison to others, a program must be utilized to help this aspect of their development. There are many strength programs available, but it is important to select one that fits the philosophy and the program.

3. Flexibility

Most coaches have limited knowledge concerning flexibility. Find a good exercise physiologist, biomechanist, gymnastic coach, or dance instructor (jazzersize or aerobics). Any of these people may help. Keep in mind that THIS IS A MUST and ask their assistance in developing a proper program if you do not have knowledge in this area.

WARNINGS AND PREVENTION

1. Double leg takedown with lift (Opponent is lifted off the mat.)

Possible injury
A. Injury to the neck region (breaks, sprains, strain)
B. Injury to shoulder area or rib cage area (break, strain)
C. Injury to offensive wrestler's back (strain, sprain)

Cause
A. Spiking opponent

B. Slamming opponent

C. Incorrect lifting technique by offensive wrestler

Prevention

A. Proper instruction as to rules, i.e., the requirement in wrestling to return opponent safely to mat.

B. Proper instruction in taking opponent back to the mat (e.g., lowering your altitude as you lower your opponent).

C. Proper instruction in using leg muscles and hip-girdle area to lift, rather than the lower back and upper body.

2. Breakdown from behind opponent when standing

Possible injury

A. Injury to shoulder and neck (fracture, strain, bruise)

B. Injury to knee (ligament, cartilage)

C. Injury to abdomen (fractured ribs, internal injuries)

Cause

A. "Tying" up opponent's near arm and tripping him toward tied-up arm.

B. Locking near leg and tripping opponent to near side.

C. Pulling opponent backward onto self.

Prevention

A. Teaching techniques that allow opponent always to protect self. (If near arm is tied up, opponent cannot protect shoulder area to tied up side.)

B. Changing rules to prohibit tying up arms on trips from behind.

C. Teaching wrestlers to trip in the direction leg flexes, not to outside where joint does not allow flexion.

D. Proper teaching technique that emphasizes the danger of bringing opponent back on self (e.g., stay higher than opponent during takedown to the mat).

3. Belly-to-belly in folkstyle and other high amplitude throws allowed in freestyle

Possible injury

A. Fractures to shoulders, neck area, or possible muscle tears or bruises

Prevention

A. Correct teaching technique that emphasizes correct procedure for the safety of both offensive and defensive wrestlers.

B. Disallowing use of high amplitude throws until wrestler is physically mature. (Need for conditioning program.)

C. Changing rules to reduce importance placed on points given for high amplitude throws (e.g., three or four points for normal takedown, one point for high amplitude throw).

4. Front or reverse stack

Possible injury
A. Fracture or strain to neck area, shoulder area, or lower back.

Cause
A. Lifting opponent at hip-girdle area and driving him forward onto neck and shoulders.
B. Lifting opponent at thigh area and driving him forward, putting pressure on lower back.

Prevention
A. Correct instruction on where not to apply pressure (e.g., neck area, lower back area).

5. Weight control

Possible injury
A. Ulcerated stomach lining, dehydration, poor electrolite balance, emotional stress, urinary tract infection, irregular bowel movements, poor endurance level causing fatigue (probably the most debilitating aspect of wrestling for all participants).

Cause
A. Inadequate instruction in weight control by coach to athletes, inadequate understanding by coach of the human body and how it functions. Too much emphasis on winning at any cost rather than learning. Inadequate record keeping of weight and weight fluctuating of athletes by coach.

Prevention
A. Training of coaches in correct method of weight control and nutrition. Emphasize to coaches and parents the need to keep up-to-date records on athletes.
B. Emphasize to coaches the safety problems with using rubber sweatsuits, saunas, steam baths.
C. Emphasize the disadvantages in use of diuretics, artificial means of weight control.

6. Maintenance of mats

Possible injury
A. Concussion

B. Neck injury

C. Staphylococus infection

Prevention

A. Checking daily, continual care, and cleaning

B. Repair of mats

C. Keep mats taped

7. Fitting and maintaining headgear

Possible injury

A. Concussion

Prevention

A. Check headgear for snug fit

B. Clean headgear periodically

C. Maintain headgear

8. Officiating

Possible injury

A. All injuries mentioned above

Prevention

A. Referee needs to be properly trained

   1. knowledge of rules

   2. experience with wrestling

   3. conditioning

   4. practice, practice, practice

B. Referees strictly enforce the rules

Part IV

Assessment, Reporting, and Litigation

29

Spacing for Safety

MARY ANN BAYLESS AND SAMUEL H. ADAMS
Washington State University
Pullman, Washington

The nature of physical education/athletics/sport/movement contains elements of danger. The level of danger is significant in some instances, almost negligible in others. Incidences range from a student moving out of place when doing a "windmill" exercise, striking another student in the eye and causing blindness, to a boy killed by being struck with a golf club, to a collision between two students while "running lines" which resulted in a permanently disabled leg.

Although a variety of literature is available which provides resource information and guidelines for prevention of serious or catastrophic injury in an activity setting, it is concentrated in the areas of facilities and equipment, correct instruction, and supervision. A conspicuously missing area of discussion in the literature, and yet one of the most important aspects of movement activities, is the area of spatial requirements for safe participation. However, a review of court cases indicates that a significant number of the injuries that result in litigation (although overall injuries are low) occur because of lack of provision for or supervision of participation with specific attention to adequate space for safe execution of the task.

Providing adequate and safe space for participation requires application of the concept of "foreseeability," which is the ability to see dangerous conditions beforehand and act to offset that danger. One application of foreseeability for teachers/coaches dictates that they must take a predictive, analytic position in order to determine appropriate organizational guidelines, develop clear and accurate instructions for student behaviors, and identify "checkpoints" with which to monitor and supervise participation. Such a predictive position allows the teacher/coach to provide well-structured practice patterns and also to be sensitive to changes in spatial relationships between individual or groups which increase the potential for injury and to respond with appropriate action.

It is understood by the authors that the guidelines for safe spacing indentified for each of the activity categories could not possibly encompass all circumstances of practice or participation. The potential for variety is too great. Neither can all activities be categorized. There is always the exception . . . or many exceptions.

The guidelines presented in this chapter are intended not only as guidelines, but also as stimulators. The careful and prudent coach and/or physical educator will attempt to foresee spacial requirements in terms of potential dangers, plan effectively to offset the dangers, and supervise in terms of both the planned provisions and predictive understanding of the potential limitations on even well-planned spatial provisions. In addition, it is hoped that the discussion will direct teachers/coaches to assess all practice activities from the perspective of foresight, (planning and supervision from knowledge of potentials), rather than respond to unforeseen circumstances.

ACTIVITIES WHICH ARE PREDOMINANTLY STATIC ALTHOUGH BODY PARTS MAY BE MOVED—NO EQUIPMENT INVOLVED

These kinds of activities include a large variety of standing, sitting, and prone exercises. Exercises may be calisthenic or warm-up activities, or activities that are part of a progression to a movement pattern or sequence of movements. Potential injury situations arise when changes in activity sequence or body position have not provided for adequate spacing. Two common problems occur. First, in all exercises that begin with a standing exercise or activity sequence, distance between participants is measured by arm reach. If the subsequent exercises require a prone or leg extension position, the original space provision may be inadequate. Second, the participant may move irregularly or off-balance during execution of exercises, requiring more space than anticipated. Many exercises, and activities in dance, martial arts, and gymnastics, require leg reach, pseudo-step, and leg extension or jump. Even though a change was not designed as part of the exercise sequence, the participant may change position (not always returning to the original starting location), creating the potential for collision with others, and/or receiving or imparting a blow to another participant.

Overall, activities in this category have a low generation of serious or catastrophic injury. However, whenever force is generated by the swinging or forceful extension of an arm or leg, potential for injury is present. The teacher/coach should consider the following guidelines during planning:

- Between-participant spacing should be determined by considering the maximum space required for any exercise, calisthenic, or movement pattern included in the exercise sequence plus an additional "buffer" space.
- Changes in how the space is being used may promote potentially dangerous circumstances and should be identified and provided for in planning.
- Students should be provided with procedures for monitoring and adjusting themselves to maintain "safe" space.
- Spatial planning should provide for unpredictable results of participation such as loss of balance or loss of control.
- Identification of potentially dangerous circumstances resulting from either changing spatial requirements or movements by an individual that carry him/her outside of his/her individual space should be part of instruction.
- Supervision should be constant and result from known difficulties or danger potentials of individual activities or movement patterns as well as the total sequence done.

ACTIVITIES THAT REQUIRE MOVEMENT FROM ONE POINT TO ANOTHER

Activities that require movement from one point to another increase the potential for serious or catastrophic injury. The participant is no longer static, but generating force as the body moves in a given direction over a given distance. The potential for injury-producing situations, as well as for severe injury, is compounded by the speed of movement, the complexity of the formation(s), and the number of individuals moving. An individual jogging for warm-up or low-level endurance training has considerably more time to respond and adjust to "unforeseen" circumstances than an individual running sprints. Running into a wall, bumping another participant, or stumbling are less likely to produce injury at slower speeds because of the decreased force produced by the slower movement.

Consideration must also be given to the formation or structure of the activity. When all participants are moving in one direction, the potential for accident is usually low. An accident can occur, however when an individual steps on another's foot, trips, jostles him/her, or misjudges passing another.

Significantly more dangerous is the situation in which participation or practice requires that individuals move in two or more directions while sharing a given space. These activities include running lines in relay situations. Any collision will have greater impact due to the force generated by bodies moving in two different directions, and significantly so at higher speeds. In relay situations, the potential for collision and injury occurs when, in the intensity of a competitive setting, the active participant runs into a waiting participant or into another competitor, either from his/her group or an adjacent group. Waiting participants, particularly toward the back of the line or group, tend to move out of line in order to watch. The active participant, concentrating on accomplishing the task, may run into an individual between lines. In running lines, collisions often occur because individuals are distracted by others and not attending to "lane" requirements, or when lanes are not clearly and distinctly identified. Also included in this category of activities are practice settings in which participants are grouped according to different activities within a larger activity category (i.e., gymnastics training stations) and must move from one practice station to another. Participants may thoughtlessly cross in front of another causing a collision. In these types of settings, equipment also infringes on the participation space as well as waiting space available to participants.

Increasing the number of participants (particularly within significant spatial limitations) multiplies the potential for collision and injury. The number of participants should be considered in applying the following guidelines.

- Identification of potentially dangerous circumstances and injuries which might result from not maintaining spatial requirements should be part of instruction.
- When all participants are moving in one direction, specific directions to be given for changing position (or limitations on changing position) should be part of the instructional planning.
- When participants are moving in two directions and sharing adjoining space, the spatial parameters or lanes for each direction should be clearly identified by verbal instruction, demonstration, and markers. Lanes should provide adequate space so that a collision will not result from a stumble or slight loss of body control.
- If the space available requires limitation on the number participating at any given time, limitations should be determined by the teacher/coach and clearly communicated to participants.
- The number of participants moving at one time and the space between participants should be controlled by the instructor, including, when necessary, signals for starting and stopping.
- If all participants are not involved in the movement pattern, space specifically assigned to "waiting" should be identified. Such space should not infringe on the area being used for movement.
- Participants not involved should not be allowed to "move casually" through the area designated for activity. Neither should they be allowed to participate in other activities which might result in an infringement, by body or piece of equipment, on the space designated for movement activity.

- Organization of relays should give special consideration to spacing requirements between lines or teams, and other non-involved individuals who might be in the immediate area (students sitting out).
- Participants should be given direct instruction on personal responsibility for alertness and maintenance of positions in lanes, specific spaces, or identified movement patterns.
- Organization should not include patterns that criss-cross unless, as in some special circumstances, practice requires it. In these instances, special safety provisions should be planned and instruction should include clear directions and procedures.

ACTIVITIES THAT REQUIRE A STRIKING ACTION

Activities in this category, which have a high potential for serious or catastrophic injury, include striking without an implement and striking with an implement. The two will be discussed separately.

Striking without an Implement

Predominant dangers in striking activities that do not require an implement can be related to being struck with a hand or fist in activities such as volleyball or handball, or a foot in activities that require kicking such as soccer and football. (The considerations of spacing related to being struck by the object is discussed in the section on propelling objects.) Being struck by a foot in the head or in an unprotected area of the body resulting in damage to an organ is probably the predominant danger, although being struck in the eye or head by an arm or fist is also a consideration. When participants are practicing, one individual may "wander" into the area being used by another participant, as when one is recovering an object or piece of equipment in order to prepare for another turn, moving to his/her own practice space, or moving to an adjacent space to wait to practice. Often these kinds of actions do not result in collision or being struck because the participant practicing is aware of the presence of another person and makes appropriate adjustment. In the instances in which injury results, however, the practicing participant may not be aware of the other person, or may judge that he/she is capable of completing the practice activity without striking the other person. Such an awareness should not be assumed as natural or the total responsibility of the participant.

Striking with an Implement

Striking activities that require an implement are innumerable and define a category of activities in which the potential for catastrophic injury is significant. This potential is present because 1) the implement usually expands the space requirement, 2) the purpose of the strike is to generate force; therefore, the swing is fast or relatively fast, and 3) the implement is usually made of a material which can inflict severe damage.

Activities that require striking with an implement fall into two sub-divisions: activities in which practice is forced around a static practice point or area, such as the golf swing or batting, and activities in which the striking action is in response to the position of another object, as in tennis or field hockey. This second sub-category results in constantly changing spatial requirements and judgmental demands on participants.

In relation to activities in which the hitting space is static, the initial requirement is to provide adequate practice space so that the implement can be swung with no possibility of interference with another participant's movements, either by striking him/her or making contact with his/her implement. The major concern then becomes that a non-practicing participant knows that he/she is present and will not swing. It is also a common tendency for participants waiting for a practice turn or moving into the waiting area to swing an implement in mock practice or in thoughtless response to having the implement in his/her hands.

Activities in which the practicing participants must respond to the path of an object and adjust the body position in order to strike it with an implement (tennis, racquetball, lacrosse, hockey, etc.) have high potential for serious or catastrophic injury. The dimensions of the space required for practice are everchanging and may be larger during one practice response than another. In addition, the situation is made more volatile when multiple hits are a part of the practice design or result from a spontaneous reaction by a participant. When more than one participant is practicing, a collision may occur, or one participant may strike the other when one participant moves to the limits of his/her space in one direction while another participant moves to the limits of his/her space in the other direction. Participants may also inadvertently "adjust" the practice space to begin at the "point of the last hit" or spot of ball retrieval rather than the original starting spot. This increases the likelihood of collision or being struck by another participant.

Non-hitting participants are, again, part of the potential for serious injury. In addition to the difficulties identified in relation to practice around a static point or area, the situation is complicated by the ever-changing spatial requirements of practice. The practicing participant may move backward to retrieve or "hit" an object and infringe on the area identified for waiting or assisting participants. This can result in collision with or striking the non-practicing participant. The condition of swinging or playing with implements (as identified in the discussion on practice from a static practice area) when in the waiting area is also a potential problem.

The teacher/coach should consider the following guidelines in planning for practice in which participants are striking, with or without an implement.

- Provision should consider the entire striking action, including preparation, follow-through, and recovery action. Any implement used for striking expands the space required for the action involved and does so in all directions around the practicing participant. In addition, the fact of the implement increases the spatial requirements for "unpredictable" results or participation. These considerations must be applied in the determination of adequate space for practice.
- Spatial designation should provide for "unpredictable" results of participation such as loss of balance or swinging and missing. This means that an additional "buffer" area be part of the practice space.
- Directions should include responsibilities of the participant and specific procedures for participant use of the practice space.
- Spatial requirements related to striking actions (with or without an implement) which require response to an object coming toward the participant should consider:
- The distance the participant is required to move to strike the object (i.e., batting a pitched ball vs. hitting a tennis forehand from a set or rebound).
- The effect on movement patterns and spatial requirements that may result from attempts at multiple hits. This is compounded when multiple hits may be done to both left and right.
- Any environmental restrictions that influence the number of participants who can practice safely (number of tennis courts, length of practice wall, racquetball court).
- Provisions should be made in planning for specifically identified space for non-practicing participants. This space should be separated from the practice space. Definition of the "waiting" space should be determined considering effects of loss of control of an implement by the practicing participant.
- Waiting participants should be given specific directions related to behaviors and alertness while in the waiting area. They should also have specific instruction on responding to practicing participants who may inadvertently move into the "waiting area."
- A specific route should be designated for entering and/or leaving the practice space which does not cut across or impinge upon the practice area of any practicing participant.

- Identified "checkpoints" to insure that movement into and out of the practice space can be done safely should be clearly communicated to participants.
- Any activity which requires that another participant be present in close proximity to the striking area (catching position for softball batting) puts additional requirements on the provision for safe use of space provided. Both the practicing participant and the other participant involved should have direct instruction on how to maintain "safe" distance.

ACTIVITIES WHICH REQUIRE THE PROPELLING OF AN OBJECT

Many sport activities require that an object be hit, thrown, kicked, or propelled, often times with an emphasis on distance and/or force as a performance requirement. Objects include those that are round, pointed, hard, soft, heavy, light, hollow, solid, and made of a variety of materials. The consequences of being struck are obvious in terms of serious or catastrophic injury, particularly if the blow involves the head, face, or unprotected body part.

In some practice settings, the participant is in a situation which dictates that an object be thrown, kicked, or struck so that it passes close or is directed toward the person practicing (baseball batting, soccer goalie, fielding in softball). The practicing individual may be struck if the object is thrown or kicked toward him/her when he/she is not ready or is distracted. Often these types of practice settings require an additional individual to back up the practicing participant a catcher or "shag." Participants involved in these roles are in a position of potential danger, either by being struck by the object or the practicing participant if adequate distance and alertness are not maintained.

Other practice settings require that the participant act from a stationary position (passing the football or throwing a ball) or after an approach (tennis stroke, javelin throw, kick). A major safety consideration in these situations is that another participant not be struck by the object propelled. Individuals not practicing may be acting as fielders, "shaggers," or chasers. Being too close to the practicing participant may result in an individual being struck because of inability to react quickly enough to a "high speed projectile." Inattention can also result in being struck, even though distance location of the individual seems appropriate. In other situations, waiting participants may "thoughtlessly" move into the area into which objects are being propelled. Sometimes a practicing participant (golf, archery) may move to recover the object or objects propelled in preparation for another turn, risking being struck.

A very dangerous situation arises when the area being used by one practicing group overlaps or is closely adjacent to another practicing group. In such situations, an object propelled by a participant in one group can strike a participant in a separate group, even though neither participant was careless or inattentive. Guidelines to be considered in developing practicing settings in which participants will be propelling objects include:

- Areas into which objects will be hit, thrown, kicked, tossed, or projected require that:

  The area be free of any other participants as the activity requires (golf, archery, shot, javelin, etc.)
  Participants performing such actions as fielding, responding, shagging, batting, or serving, should be adequate distances away to react to the objects.

- Spatial requirements should be determined considering that the object may not always go in the direction intended by the practicing participant. In these situations, the size and weight of the object as well as the striking action have implications for spatial determination.
- When several participants are practicing at one time, the space into which objects are being propelled should not overlap another practicing participant or the space into which objects are being propelled of another practice group. An additional "buffer" space should be provided between practicing groups.
- If some coordination of propelling an object and returning the object to the initiator or some specified point is required, planning must include provision for free space around and in line with any and all target points. (Returning objects to the location of the practicing participant may require planning for safe use of space as much as the act being practiced.)
- If practice includes the collection of objects thrown, kicked, struck, propelled, or shot, there must be provision for control of participant movement and entry into the area into which objects have been propelled.
- Specific instructions for all participants, in terms of all of the requirements for practice and the safe use of space, should be identified and clearly communicated.

OTHER FACTORS

The guidelines presented in this chapter have not specifically applied the consideration of the age, maturity, skill level, conditioning, and number of participants in an activity. However, these considerations are of the utmost importance in "foreseeing" potential dangers related to spacing. Professional competence in knowledge and ability to utilize knowledge to make judgments is essential. In other words, a teacher/ coach must not only know proper technique and proper spatial requirements in the activity being conducted, but should also know and understand the biological and psychological qualitites of the participants and their relationship to the activity being taught. Maturity, skill level, and conditioning have great significance for planning progression, deciding how much and how strict supervision should be, detail of instruction, and sequencing of activities. (It is obvious that a thorough knowledge of all of these characteristics of participants—age, maturity, skill level, conditioning, and number participating in the activity influence spatial requirements.)

Baley and Matthews (1984) point out the importance of knowing participants in regard to age, knowledge, judgment, and experience by identifying how courts in most states view the individual participant's contributory negligence.

> In most states a child under the age of majority is bound to exercise such care for his own safety as would ordinarily be exercised by a child of like age, knowledge, judgement, and experience under the facts, circumstances and conditions disclosed by the evidence. It therefore becomes incumbent upon the coach, teacher, or person in charge to give explicit instructions. To ensure that these instructions are actually communicated to the children or persons involved, they should be posted on signs or handed out in printed or mimeographed form.

They state again:

> The coach has a duty to be aware of the background and experience of the participants, and to be personally familiar with the ability of participants.

In the *Diker vs. City of St. Louis Park,* 130 N.W. 2nd 113, the Minnesota Supreme Court stated:

> Children, through childish in-attention, may fail to observe conditions which an adult might reasonably be expected to discover. Even if they know of the condition, there may be risks which it may not be reasonable to assume that children will appreciate.

Leibee (1965) points out that some courts, when looking at the assumption of risk for which a child may be held accountable, use a method which requires looking into the child's experience, background, capacity (intelligence), and age. A professional coach/teacher will, therefore, be held to a competence level that will make them cognizant of these characteristics in the students they teach and coach.

In terms of spacing, this adds another dimension for coaches/teachers to consider. All guidelines will have to be more careful and detailed in explanation and demonstration. Repetition of guidelines to students is imperative. The guidelines should be written and displayed. Supervision of activities will have to be more closely monitored. Foreseeability on the part of the teacher will have to be carefully considered when the students have less responsibility for their actions.

30

Action Model to Evaluate and Reduce Risk of Catastrophic Injuries

Marlene Adrian
University of Illinois Urbana-Champaign
Urbana-Champaign, Illinois

A fundamental approach to the investigation of catastrophic injuries is the formulation of a plan of action or model (Figure 30- 1) for assessment of risk of catastrophic injury. Such a model should consist of the identification of all components of the sports situation. One may then analyze each component with respect to aspects of risk and magnitude of risk of catastrophic injury.

The model depicted in Figure 30-1 represents the components without the details of component analysis. Thus the teacher, coach and athletic administrator need to address the characteristics of the players, the sport itself, the external environment of the sport, and the health support services with respect to each particular sport. The analysis of the major components of the model results in the identification of potential risks and a plan of action for reducing these risks. This plan of action includes proposed changes in some aspect of one or more of these components. Each component will be discussed in the following pages. Each one of these components will be scrutinized and the process of isolating the risk factors will be presented.

No matter how many years one has taught or coached players in a particular sport, this scrutinization process should be performed at the beginning of the season or course of study, as well as at selected points during the period of play. The analogy may be made to the procedures each pilot of an airplane follows step-by-step with a cue card prior to each take-off, no matter how many times the pilot has flown that particular airplane. One cannot be too careful with respect to procedures for evaluation of potential risk of catastrophic injury.

Figure 30-1. Catastrophic Injury Assessment

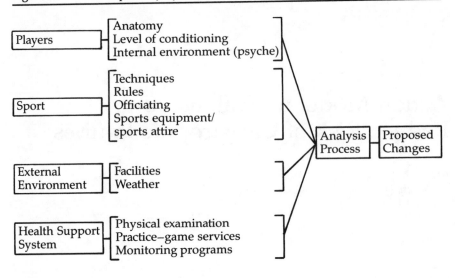

THE PLAYERS

The factors to be examined in this section are portrayed in (Table 30-1). Foremost in the assessment of possible risk to players is consideration of morphological characteristics of the players. Are they homogeneous with respect to size, weight, and height? What is the relative muscle-weight ratio for each player? Are the players very young or very old, thus potentially high-risk individuals? Are some of the players physically or mentally handicapped? A person without impairment of limbs or nervous system will be able to avert a catastrophic injury more easily than will one with a physical impairment. In general, the greater the differences among the group of players, the greater will be the possibility of the smallest and lightest being injured by the largest and heaviest if contact is involved. Likewise, the level of skill of each individual will influence the speeds at which the players will move. The greater the speed and the greater the mass, the greater will be the risk of injury during a collision.

In addition, the level of conditioning of each player needs to be assessed. Catastrophic injuries may occur during the fatigued state and consequent collisions and falls by these fatigued players. The teacher and coach should know the minimal requirements in strength, speed, and balance for a player to participate safely in the sport. Individualized physical conditioning programs need to be designed to produce these minimal requirements, plus a margin of safety. These programs will also reduce the heterogeneity of the players and improve their status for play.

Table 30-1. The Players

Morphological/Mechanical Characteristics	Internal State	Action for Change
Larger size		Providing pre-season and in-season conditioning
Strong		
Fast in movement skills		Selecting optimal playing position
High in muscle/weight ratio	No anxiety	
Skilled	Low anxiety	Providing proper education and skill development
Well-conditioned	Optimal anxiety	
Poor-conditioned	High competitive anxiety	Matching for sizes during practice
Unskilled		Regulating forces in practice
Symptoms of previous injuries or unhealthy condition	Fearful of situation	Individualizing physical conditioning programs
Weak		Providing extra protection
Lean in muscle/weight ratio		Elimination from team
Small size		

The internal states of the players may, however, be more important than their outward characteristics. Players who are overly fearful of a situation or have greater than optimum anxiety when confronted with certain situations within the sport are prime targets for injury. Strategies need to be devised for achieving an optimum psychological state within each player prior to play and maintaining this state during play.

Therefore the approach in coaching a group of players will change with respect to each group of players. The progression and, indeed, the emphases, will vary with respect to the group and the individuals within the group. In Table 30-1 there are several action plans for changing the characteristics of the players or adjusting to the existing characteristics. The broad categories encompassed in this figure include the following:

1. Profiling each player
2. Individualizing instruction
3. Individualizing conditioning programs
4. Controlling the forces in practice and game situations
5. Eliminating the players from the team

The systematic and synthesized presentation of characteristics of each player is termed profiling. It is by means of profiling that the coach is able to understand the unique strengths and weaknesses of each player. Common characteristics and homogeniety can also be identified. Therefore the coach (and teacher of sports classes) must test and measure the players, not only on skills of the sport but on basic anatomy and movement abilities. It is especially important with young athletes to discover physical anomalies that can be corrected early. Many sports organizations, including the U.S. Olympic Committee, have become interested in the concepts of profiling. The International Society of Biomechanics in Sports has made this a major emphasis. Publications on this topic by Anjos and Adrian appear in the references.

THE SPORT

Each sport has a number of techniques for play. Special attention must be given to those techniques in which collisions occur, high acceleration rates are produced, and the human body is oriented other than upright in space. Practice, conditioning, and a thorough understanding of the mechanics of these techniques are vital to protecting the player and eliminating undue risk.

The following questions should be asked about each sport:
1. Is there body contact among the players?
2. Does the body contact involve the head, neck, or trunk?
3. Would body contact produce a collision that would cause loss of equilibrium with probable landing on the head, neck, or trunk?
4. If there is no body contact among the players, could any situation during play cause collisions with other objects, including the ground, that would produce loss of equilibrium?

Answers of yes to one or more of these questions requires that the possibility of a catastrophic injury be considered. Thus one must evaluate the probability factor. For example, loss of equilibrium and severe injury are most apt to happen in situations in which the speeds prior to the collision, the maximal forces at impact, and the displacement of the line of gravity of the body with respect to the base of support are the greatest.

Familiarity with the research concerning collisions and forces and subsequent injuries involved in the sports situation provides a foundation from which to develop teaching and coaching strategies. Conditioning programs can be scientifically developed specific to the forces encountered in the sport. If one cannot condition sufficiently, the sports attire and equipment may be modified or protective equipment may be worn. New and modified techniques and changes in the rules of the game are also possibilities to consider.

One of the major considerations in maintaining safety and thus averting catastrophic injury is to use equipment that meets national standard specifications. There are three major types of governing bodies involved in writing standards for products used in sports: government agencies, professional organizations, and open member organizations.

The Consumer Product Safety Commission is the government agency responsible for consumer products in the United States. The American Society for Testing of Materials (ASTM) and the American National Standards Institute are the comparable open membership organizations. Professional organizations include such committees as the National Operating Committee on Standards for Athletic Equipment, which writes standards only in sports and only in the area of head and neck equipment, and the Hockey Equipment Certification Council of the Amateur Hockey Association of the United States, which is specific to one sport but all equipment in that sport. There is cooperation and often joint efforts in developing common standards among all these organizations.

The most comprehensive organization for standards in sports equipment and facilities is ASTM since it has technical subcommittees on padding, playing surfaces, head gear, eye protection, football, wrestling, ski safety, fencing, footwear, female athletes, archery, equestrian, playground surfaces, fitness and health, and medical aspects of sports. Consumers, manufacturers, and general interest persons (including biomechanics researchers) actively cooperate to develop national voluntary consensus standard practices, definitions, test methods, classifications, and specifications concerning sports equipment and facilities. A listing of activities of these committees and the standards which have been produced through ASTM can be obtained by writing to the ASTM-Sports Equipment and Facilities F.8 Committee in Philadelphia.

Selected plans of action for preventing catastrophic injuries are listed in Table 30-2. These are guidelines for the analysis of each sport; action must be specific to the sport.

THE EXTERNAL ENVIRONMENT

The external environment consists of the playing surface, designated structures, and non-playing area. Each presents no risk of catastrophic injury if it complies with the specifications of the rule book of that sport. Weather and lighting, as well as lack of compliance with standard specifications, will change the level of safety of this external environment. Thus the coach and teacher must decide whether or not to cancel practice or the game, should playing become dangerous. Modifications might be made in footwear, especially when the playing surface is frozen, wet, or muddy.

The structures may need to be padded and rules of play modified for non-compliance situations. Inadequate non-playing areas and obstructions outside the playing area pose unsafe conditions. Table 30-3 presents an example for assessing and improving the external environment.

Table 30-2. The Sport

Component	Characteristics	Action for Change
Techniques of game	Collisions Accelerations	Know and understand mechanics of techniques
	Orientation of body in space	Take precautions for situations placing players in inverted positions Condition for these techniques
Rules of game	Safety items	Read rules, know them Address safety items
Officiating	Practice Competition	Insist upon proper officiating at all times
Sports equipment	Weights Physical dimensions Rigidity Durability Elasticity	Use equipment that meets national standards Report inadequate equipment to manufacturers Communicate with ASTM F.8
Sports facility	Obstructions Playing surface Dimensions Surroundings	Evaluate prior to each use, correct problems
Sports attire	Special protective devices Regular body covering	Evaluate adequacy, including fit

HEALTH SUPPORT SYSTEM

The health support system (Table 30-4) includes the pre-season physical examination, at which time spinal cord/spinal column abnormalities can be identified. Prior histories of head and heart anomalies can be assessed with respect to risk of participation in selected sports.

Based upon the evaluation of the other major components of the action model to evaluate and reduce risk of catastrophic injuries, the type and amount of practice-and-game-time health services can be determined. The coach or some other designated person should be knowledgeable in first aid and trained to perform correctly in situations in which head, neck, or trunk injury is known or suspected to have occurred. A potentially catastrophic injury may be converted to a minor injury through proper on-site procedures, or the original injury can be compounded by incorrect treatment.

A desirable support system includes a system for monitoring the players, their condition state, injury status, and other characteristics.

Table 30-3. External Environment

Component	Characteristics	Action for Change
Playing surface	Weather changes caused: ice, moisture, freeze, cracks, mud, buckling, etc.	Evaluate surface/risk of injury Decision to play or not play Modify footwear Modify playing surface Change location
Visibility	Lighting is insufficient to see designated structures, players	Evaluate response deficit and risk of injury Decision to play or not play Modify color of ball
Playing facility	Does not meet safety standards	Modify rules of play Evaluate required changes

Table 30-4. Health Support System

Components	Output Characteristics	Action for Change
Physical Examination	Identification of risk	"Bench" player
Practice-game services	Training in what to do if head, neck, and trunk injured. Personnel with knowledge of first-aid	Medical consultation concerning adequacy of services
Monitoring programs	Data bank of injuries Data bank of conditioning sessions	Modify schedule, practice, or equipment if any are suspected of contributing to injury

Such a system represents a preventative measure against the unforeseen. One may be able to anticipate a catastrophe, thus averting it.

For further information concerning assessment of safety and risk of injury, the reader is referred to the Sports Safety Series of AAHPERED, and especially the 1977 article by Adrian and Klinger. Safety requires constant surveillance of the total sports arena. Administrators of sports programs can assist the coach in many ways, especially in the facilitation of facility maintenance, equipment purchasing, and health support systems organization. The sport and the players, however, are primarily the daily responsibility of the coach.

31

Catastrophic Injury Surveillance and Reporting

The following is reprinted from: Fourth Annual National Gymnastic Catastrophic Injury Report, 1981-1982; *Copyright 1983 by the United States Gymnastics Safety Association, Vienna, VA. Reprinted by permission.*

BACKGROUND

Football has been the only school/college sport from which catastrophic injury data have been collected over the years. Since 1931, the Annual Survey of Football Fatalities of the American Football Coaches Association (in cooperation with the National Collegiate Athletic Association and the National Federation of State High School Associations) has followed the trends of *fatal* injuries in organized football as the nature of that game changed over the years. In 1975, the National Football Head and Neck Injury Registry was initiated by the Philadelphia Sports Medicine Center (in cooperation with the National Athletic Trainers Association) to make *nonfatal* catastrophic injuries (e.g., quadriplegia) an equally understood concern. Thanks to the continuity of these endeavors, not only have preventive efforts been formulated and implemented based on the observed trends, but an effectiveness of these efforts has been observed as well.

Football is not the only sport associated with the occasional occurrence of a catastrophic injury. A survey of catastrophic sports injuries in high schools and colleges nationally from 1973 through 1975 found Gymnastics to have had a higher average annual relative frequency than football. Wrestling also showed an annual persistence of such injuries, but only Gymnastics and Football presented the describable patterns of injury which are needed to guide preventive efforts.

The label "Gymnastics" encompasses a diversity of activities and apparatuses. Predominantly implicated with the reported gymnastic catastrophic injuries was the trampoline (although not to the exclusion of other gymnastic activities). Subsequently, in 1977, the American Academy of Pediatrics (AAP) publicly warned against the use of the trampoline. In 1978, the American Alliance for Health, Physical Education, Recreation, and Dance (AAHPERD) issued guidelines for the controlled use of the trampoline and minitramp in physical education and cheerleading (Appendix B), as did the NCAA Committee on Competitive Safeguards and Medical Aspects of Sports for the trampoline's use as a training device by skilled athletes (Appendix C). In 1981, a revision of the 1977 American Academy of Pediatrics (AAP) was published (Appendix D).

These Guidelines emerged from an analysis of the circumstances associated with the catastrophic trampoline and minitramp injury reports available from the 1973-1975 survey, the U.S. Consumer Product Safety Commission, and gymnastic equipment manufacturers. Essentially, the vast majority of catastrophic injuries stemmed from improper landings *on* the trampoline from poorly executed somersaults, while the catastrophic minitramp injuries resulted from either poorly executed multiple somersault attempts or movement of the minitramp at takeoff. These Gudelines have been shared in draft with representatives of allied organizations in preparation for open hearings on the eve of the AAHPERD National Convention in April 1978. The hearing were well attended (e.g., U.S. Gymnastics Safety Association, President's Council on Physical Fitness and Sport, National Safety Council, American Academy of Pediatrics) with support clearly the concensus expression of that group. Three days later, the AAHPERD Assembly formally adopted the guidelines for physical education and extended the support of the NCAA guidelines being considered for varsity athletes. The NCAA Committee adopted their guidelines at their semiannual meeting in June 1978.

These guidelines succinctly identify the essential safety prerequisites for those who wish to pursue the benefits of trampolining and those who provide administrative and actuarial support of these programs. The recommended implementation plans included widespread publicity of the guidelines among AAHPERD member, school and college administrators, coaches, insurance carriers, and allied organizations. In addition, experts on trampolining were encouraged to write professional articles on the "how to" aspects of the statements' intents. The next step was to begin monitoring the subsequent nature and frequency of catastrophic injuries from trampolining and other gymnastic activities.

THE NATIONAL GYMNASTIC
CATASTROPHIC INJURY REGISTRY

Serious head-neck-spine injuries had been found to occur infrequently yet persistently in gymnastics, and reliable data were needed to characterize the patterns and relative frequency of such injuries on a continuous basis. Being infrequent, such data have to be pooled from the entire nation's experiences to have meaning and to assess with confidence the effectiveness of particular preventive measures. The National Gymnastic Catastrophic Injury Registry was conceived to this end in Spring 1978 while AAHPERD and NCAA were pursuing the adoption of their safety guidelines for trampoline and minitramp use in physical education and sport. Subsequently, the U.S. Gymnastics Safety Association agreed to serve as its principal sponsor, with the Registry Office maintained at the University of Illinois and supported by initiation grants from AMF, GAS Athletic Equipment, Nissen Corporation, and Porter Equipment Company.

The objective of the Registry is to collect information on every permanent neurological injury (spinal cord or cerebral, fatal or nonfatal) in the nation resulting from a gymnastic accident, including cheerleading, effective July 1, 1978. The purpose is to report annually on the frequency of such serious injuries and to the apparent patterns of injury which may lead to preventive measures. The annual report is to also include, on occasion, information being collected on less serious yet significant gymnastic injuries reported to the National Athletic Injury/Illness Reporting System (NAIRS) and other sources of relevant information.

The goals of the Registry were readily feasible because of the variety of national organizations sharing responsibility for the offering of gymnastic and cheerleading who agreed to serve as cosponsors:

American Academy of Pediatrics
American College Health Association
American School and Community Safety Association
Association for Intercollegiate Athletics for Women
National Association of Collegiate Directors of Athletics
National Association of Intercollegiate Athletics
National Cheerleader Coaches' Association
National Collegiate Athletic Association
National Council of YMCA's
National Federation of State High School Associations
National Junior College Athletic Association
National Parks and Recreation Association
National Safety Council

Society of State Directors of Health, Physical Education
and Recreation
United States Association of Independent Gymnastics Clubs
United States Cheerleaders Association
United States Gymnastics Federation
United States Gymnastics Safety Association

(The following is reprinted from 1981).

U.S. CONSUMER PRODUCT SAFETY REPORT

A recent study by (December, 1981) the U.S. Consumer Product Safety Commission entitled "Overview of Sports-Related Injuries to Persons 5-14 Years of Age" found a decline in the number of head and neck trampoline injuries reported through NEISS (National Electronic Injury Surveillance System) by almost two-thirds since 1978 (1,755 to 600). This number of 600 is not catastrophic injuries, but general head and neck injuries. They did, however, find head and neck injuries stayed about the same in general for other sports as it had been in the past.

It is also interesting to note some of their other relevant findings with regards to gymnastics. The 1981 "Overview of Sports-Related Injuries to Persons 5-14 Years of Age" also reported that:

> Overall, children 5-14 sustain 31 percent of the sports-related injuries. The sports examined with the highest proportion of victims in this age group were tetherball and gymnastics. Those with the lowest proportions in the 5-14 age group were racquetball, lacrosse, and volleyball.

Again, it needs to be stressed this is for injuries in general, and *not* catastrophic injuries. We are using the definition of catastrophic injuries as those that result in permanent paralysis as a paraplegic or quadriplegic.

Regarding fatalities in this same report, the study found "more fatalities of children resulted from the child being struck by a ball or puck in a game, than from any other scenario." They found with their research that "two-thirds (62 of 94) of the sports related deaths reported involved injury from impact with a secondary object like a baseball, bat, golf club, hockey stick, or puck . . . Baseball fatalities to children 5-14 were surprisingly high, and the baseball injury and fatality data warrant further investigation and analysis."

Because of the importance of the findings in the "Overview of Sports-Related Injuries to Persons 5-14 Years of Age," parts of the report will be given below as it explains more clearly the scope and depth of their research findings:

This report deals with a group of 15 selected sports activities. During 1980, there were 1.8 million medically attended injuries to persons 5-14 years of age, related to participation in these activities. Nearly 600,000 of these persons were treated in hospital emergency rooms. Reports of 105 fatalities associated with the same group of sports were received by the Consumer Product Safety Commission. (During the 8 year period from 1973 through 1980.)

The dual purposes of the report were to provide an overview of available sports-related injury data involving children, and to identify injury trends or sports activities worthy of further examination from an injury perspective. The sports included in this report were: football, baseball, basketball, gymnastics, soccer, wrestling, volleyball, ice hockey, track and field, racquet sports, golf, trampoline, tetherball, lacrosse, and other ball sports.

More specifically, it is of interest to look at the Sports-Related Medically Attended Injuries to Persons 5-14 Years of Age:

The report focuses on sports-related injuries to children 5-14 years of age. The sports activities reviewed were chosen because children of this age frequently participate in these activities, particularly in a school or other organized environment. More than 5 million medically attended injuries to persons of all ages are associated with the sports included in this report.

A list of the sports selected and an estimate of the number of medically attended injuries to persons 5-14 years of age associated with each during 1980 is on the following page. Also shown is the number of deaths in the age group reported to the Consumer Product Safety Commission (CPSC) for each sport activity over the 8 year period from 1973 through 1980.

Looking at this report more closely with regards to fatalities, there were *no* fatalities reported for gymnastics, volleyball, or lacrosse, but there were 6 in trampoline. The other sports that had fatalities included: baseball (40), football (19), golf (13), ball (nos) (7), basketball (6), soccer (6), track and field (2), wrestling (2), ice hockey (2), racquet sports (1), tetherball (1), for a total of 105 fatalities.

Table 1A: Sports-Related Medically Attended Injuries to Persons 5-14 Years of Age During Calendar Year 1980, and Fatalities January 1973-December 1980

Sport	Medically Attended Injuries[2]	Deaths
Total	1,800,500	105
Football	499,400	19
Baseball	359,400	40
Basketball	295,300	6
Gymnastics	209,200	0
Ball Sports, N.O.S.[3]	133,200	7
Soccer	107,400	6
Wrestling	55,100	2
Volleyball	46,500	0
Ice Hockey	28,900	2
Track and Field	22,600	2
Racquet Sports	17,100	1
Golf	11,600	13
Trampoline	7,200	6
Tetherball	5,500	1
Lacrosse	2,100	0

[2] Estimates of medically attended injuries are derived by multiplying estimates of emergency room-treated injuries by factors based on the National Center for Health Statistics, Health Interview Survey. Estimates of emergency room treated injuries are from the National Electronic Injury Surveillance System (NEISS).

[3] Ball Sports, N.O.S.—This category includes injuries associated with sports for which the specific activity was not reported.

IMPLICATIONS OF THESE TWO REPORTS

The previously cited data represent injuries in unsupervised sports situations, as well as in organized sport situations. No causes have been identified, and few details of each incident are given. Thus it is evident that teachers and coaches need to monitor catastrophic injuries and to be aware of catastrophic injuries occurring in sports. Each teacher and coach should contribute to the reduction of catastrophic injuries by sharing information, developing or maintaining an existing registry of catastrophic injuries, and reading safety research. The National Athletic Injury Reporting System (NAIRS) has a small data bank from high schools and colleges/universities that is worth investigation. The American Society for Testing of Materials (ASTM) FO.8 Committee personnel rely heavily upon injury data to determine requirements for standards. Unfortunately, such data often are lacking.

The development of minimum standards in the area of knowledge of safety is one approach to assure qualified teachers and coaches. The United States Gymnastic Federation (USGF) has established a certification program for instructors of gymnastics. In addition, the federation has published a gymnastics safety manual (see References, USGF 1985) that is being used as the text for their safety certification program. Other sports associations may determine that such a program is useful for their sports.

Officiating organizations also have been leaders in promoting safety in sports competition. For example, the Associated Board of Officials of the National Association for Girls and Women in Sport was organized to standardize and improve the caliber of officiating nationwide. Today this officiating organization conducts the most comprehensive and stringent training sessions in the sports of basketball and volleyball. Trained, certified, or otherwise qualified officials should be secured for all competitive events. Coaches must support those officials who control the game, albeit stringently, and cooperate in the elimination of "lax" officiating.

Coaches, administrators, and other leaders and teachers of sports have an obligation to assist the sports governing bodies for rules and policies. This can be done by responding to questionnaires and cooperating in the evaluation of new and proposed rule changes. In addition, these personnel may initiate a plea for changes in rules.

The information in this book comprises the minimum safety information in sports. This book, therefore, could be the basis for examination of minimum certification for safety in coaching.

32

Summary of Litigation In Physical Education and Sport*

ANNIE CLEMENT
Cleveland State University
Cleveland, Ohio

Physical educators and coaches have become increasingly concerned about the possibility of being named in law suits. Connors (1981) and Appenzeller (1978) note that physical educators and coaches are the persons most often sued in the educational setting. Connors (1978, p. 1X) in Educational Tort Liability and Malpractice,

> estimates that one-third of the suits brought against educators are settled out of court in the U.S., because the teachers were so obviously negligent that the insurance companies involved did not want to face juries. I also estimate that approximately one-third of the suits brought against educators are routinely dismissed by trial judges as being trivial, because the teachers were obviously not negligent. That leaves about 33% of the suits resulting in jury trials where the issue of negligence is real. Of that number, about one-half are appealed. There are between 200 and 500 appealed cases reported every year; this means that there are probably between 1,200 and 3,000 suits brought against teachers or administrators every year.

DEFINITION

A tort is an injury proximately caused by breach of a legal duty; a tort exists when an injury occurs as a result of someone's failure to honor

---

*Substantial portions of this chapter have been taken from Educational Malpractice; Physical Educators Should be Concerned, *The Physical Educator* (in press).

a legal duty. Among the duties of the physical educator are the duty to inspect equipment for safety and the duty to provide instruction appropriate to the student's level of skills.

The three basic types of tort are intentional torts, such as battery; strict liability torts, such as engaging in extra hazardous activities; and injuries caused by negligent behavior (Keeton, 1984, p. 1-5). An act will be considered negligent when all of the following elements are present:

1. A duty of care (or legal duty as mentioned above) must exist and must be owed to the person injured.
2. The duty of care must have been breached.
3. Injury must be as a result of the breach of the duty of care.
4. Damage has to have occurred.

In educational malpractice, for example, faulty teaching or the use of faulty tests may result in injury. The injury or damage to the student is failure to learn or failure to be able to obtain a job. In physical education and sport, failure to learn a skill may also result in a physical injury. If a teacher failed to provide adequate instruction to a student who is ready to dive from a diving board, the student may sustain a physical injury as he/she enters the water. Such an injury could be a result of malpractice or the failure to properly instruct.

CONTEMPORARY PHYSICAL EDUCATION

An examination of contemporary physical education cases provides specific instructions for the teacher. In *Lueck v. City of Janesville* (1973), the court found no evidence that the teacher had failed to use ordinary care in furnishing adequate equipment or in the instruction, supervision, or assistance given to the student. The plaintiff, 17-year-old high school student, was attempting to do a forward roll on still rings when he slipped and fell, sustaining serious injuries. A summary of how the competent teacher in this situation testified follows:

1. Provided student's grades for the past two years and the criteria upon which they were derived.
2. Identified the progression used in teaching gymnastics and the level of difficulty of the stunt the student was performing at the time of the accident.
3. Verified that instruction had been provided sufficient to enable the student to describe the skill level of the stunt and precautions requisite to its successful performance. Students were also able to take the stand and attest to the details of instruction.
4. Clearly articulated his approach to individualized instruction.
5. Student and teacher provided detailed descriptions of the safety procedures used in progressions, in determining student's capacity to perform, and in assessing the need for a spotter. Fur-

ther, plaintiff/student knew and could relate to the court the fact that he was not to execute a new stunt without going over it with the instructor.

6. Competent expert witnesses explained individualized instruction in gymnastics and the value of its use in the classroom. They also addressed the topic of spotting and its relationship to the acquisition of self confidence.

7. In response to the alleged negligence of the teacher in failing to assign a spotter to a performing student, the expert and the defendant demonstrated that there were no facts to support negligence but that the idea of the need for a spotter at all times was speculative.

The standard of care in this situation was the standard of a reasonable physical educator. Although professionals might have higher personal standards, when they choose to serve as expert witnesses they must work with standards that are reasonable. The Lueck case is highly instructive to the well-organized, motivated teacher and particularly helpful to the creative teacher whose class organization and teaching progression might not meet the evidence standard of a traditional program. It appeared to the writer than Lueck was upheld because his planning was thorough, he engaged counsel who believed in the capability of the client, and he was able to articulate his goals and demonstrate that he was, in fact, a competent teacher.

In *Larson v. Independent School District No. 314 Brahan* (1979), an eighth grade student became a quadriplegic after breaking his neck while performing a handspring over a rolled mat. The first-year teacher, with one month of experience on the job, was found negligent in the spotting and teaching of the exercise. The case provided the following facts which the reader should note.

1. Curriculum bulletins used by the Minnesota district as a standard for planning and teaching were considered relevant in the jury determination of whether defendant had breached his duty of care. Such bulletins were not to be considered mandatory affirmative requirements; however, in situations where the bulletins were not used, the teacher was expected to identify the conceptual plan to which he was committed.

2. The principal had responsibility for informing a new teacher of his/her duties.

3. The principal was responsible for an examination of the progression for, in this case, gymnastics and a determination of whether the teacher was executing the steps as traditionally used. One specific question asked was whether an advanced skill had been introduced to the student before it could be ascertained that the student knew the elementary skills?

4. Proper spotting or adequate safety devices unique to the activity were documented as used in the classroom.
5. Unit plans existed and were produced. The expert witness stressed the need for detailed unit and lesson planning for beginning teachers. Unit planning was considered essential to ensure proper progression and safety.
6. It was deemed essential that substitutes and new teachers become aware of each student's capacity with reference to baseline skills.

Although the physical educator was found liable, a reading of the case points out the exact reasons for the court's decision and can serve to guide physical educators in preparing plans and in defending their programs. What this case established was that where a well-planned physical education program existed and could be documented, the courts were eager to support the teacher. In situations where planning was inadequate, the courts found it difficult to support the professional. Although the case does not deal with the situation in which the planning was adequate but the documentation was inadequate, one can recognize the problems that would exist in providing evidence to the court in such a situation. While documentation is vital, professionals should remember that competent planning and skillful execution of instruction is the framework upon which a successful defense is built and documented.

A situation in which a student obtained a verdict for damage to her mouth as a result of an injury sustained when she was taught a preliminary run as part of the jump and reach test in found in *Dibortolo v. Metropolitan School District* (1982). Expert testimony verified that instruction for the jump and reach test required that a student begin in a standing, not a running position. The court said,

> the evidence that [the teacher] did not demonstrate the exercise, that she specifically directed the student to run during a structured physical activity such as the vertical jump, when juxtaposed with the expert testimony, that such an instruction is not only erroneous, but is also unsafe, would have entitled a jury to reasonably infer that the teacher's conduct exposed the student to an unreasonable risk. Furthermore, there was sufficient evidence from which a jury could have justifiably concluded that [the teacher's] instructions were the proximate cause of the plaintiff's injury. A proximate cause of plaintiff's injury is one which sets in motion the chain of circumstances leading to the injury. (p. 511)

A recent case in which the teacher's instruction was upheld was *Smith v. Vernon Parish School Board* (1983). A 15-year-old straight "A" student was injured when she joined four other students in jumping on a trampoline while the teacher had briefly left the room. Student testimony established that the students had been instructed not to jump in a group or to jump without supervision and that while executing the feat they had assigned one of their group to hide in the curtains of the stage and keep an eye on the whereabouts of the teacher. This case not only reinforced the need to provide proper instruction to students but gave support for the principle that when the instruction was adequate the teacher's presence in the gymnasium may not be necessary. What was important was that the instruction had been given and that each student who testified knew of the instruction and was able to repeat the instruction while on the stand.

SUMMARY OF ELEMENTS TO CONSIDER IN PROGRAM PLANNING AND CURRICULAR REFORM

1. Physical educators should recognize the following general concepts:
   A. Many injuries are sustained in physical education; therefore, professionals are vulnerable to litigation (Korpela, 1985, p. 364).
   B. The courts are more inclined to make a decision in a case involving a physical injury than they are in one involving a psychological injury.
   C. Courses of study, curriculum bulletins, and lesson plans must be available, must document learning and progression, and must be introduced as evidence.
   D. Adequate information should be available with reference to each student's skill capacity to enable the teacher to justify the physical demand placed on a particular student.
   E. When instructions are given and repeated, the majority of the members of any class, if placed on the stand, should be able to verify that such instructions were given.
   F. Whatever methodology is employed for instruction—demonstration, film, or verbal cue—it must meet the test of peer scrutiny. Whenever an unorthodox technique or strategy is used, the teacher should be aware of professionals who would support the approach. No teacher should be forced into a particular approach, progression or teaching strategy; however, each teacher should be able to readily explain why a particular approach was used on a specific day.
2. Concepts specific to the coaching of sports should be fully understood. They include:

A. Official rules are to be obeyed when their use is appropriate to the learning situation.
B. Players are to be warned of possible catastrophic injuries. They and their parents are to be informed of potential risk of catastrophic injury, even though the risk is low.
C. Players are to be informed that protective equipment does not prevent the occurrence of a catastrophic injury, but only reduces the probability of a catastrophic injury.
D. Coaches and teachers are to use instructional strategies designed to prevent catastrophic injuries.
E. Risk management strategies should govern the decision to eliminate known situations that might cause injury.
F. Knowledge of certification, injuries, data systems, and safety precautions is to be sought.
G. Communication among bodies that set sports standards (i.e., the American Society for Testing of Materials F.8 committee), governing associations, officiating bodies, competitive sports governing organizations, coaches, and sports administrators must exist.
H. Special safety precautions should be taken with respect to:
   1. Collisions
   2. Projectiles and swinging objects (balls, sticks)
   3. Aerial activities
   4. Natural elements (lightning, heat, sun)
I. All head, neck, and trunk injuries must be treated as potential catastrophes. Don't believe the athlete! Be conservative.
J. Compliance with standards for equipment and facilities must not be compromised.
K. Identify anomalies among athletes, and use medical help to screen for problems.
L. Prepare the players, physically and mentally, for the sport. Comprehensive planning and execution of the plan should enable any teacher to go to court with confidence. Planning is essential to ensure competent teaching and coaching, accountability, ease of instruction, and last but not least, the provision of a learning environment in which the teacher or coach can easily establish a defense or an explanation for any activity which ultimately could be questioned by a court of law.

References

Aaron, J.E., ed.
    1979   *First Aid and Emergency Care*. Second Edition. New York: MacMillan Publishing Co.

Adams, S.
    1982   Court Decision Hits Hard with New Liability Twists. *Athletic Purchasing and Facilities* 7:12.
    1984   Liability and the Physical Educator. *The Physical Educator* 41(4): 200-204.

Adams, S., M. Adrian, and M.A. Bayless, eds.
    1984   *Catastrophic Injuries in Sports—Avoidance Strategies*. Salinas, CA: Coyote Press.

Adams, S, and M.A. Bayless
    1982   Clear, Specific Instruction is your Best Position. *Athletic Purchasing and Facilities*, August.

Adrian, M., and A. Klinger
    1977   Field Hockey. In: *Safety in Team Sports*, J. Borozne, C.A. Morehouse, and S.F. Pechar, eds. Washington, D.C.: AAHPER Publications.

American Red Cross
    1973   *Lifesaving, Rescue and Water Safety*. Garden City, New York: Doubleday and Co.
    1974   *Lifesaving, Rescue and Water Safety*. Washington, D.C.: The American Red Cross.

American Society for the Testing of Materials (ASTM)
    1. ANSI/ASTM F513-81 Eye and Face Protective Equipment for Hockey Players. Philadelphia.
    2. ANSI/ASTM F697-80 Standard Practice for Care and Use of Mouth Guards. Philadelphia.
    3. Committee on Sports Equipment and Facilities, Minutes of Ice Hockey Subcommittee Meetings: April, 1979; October, 1982; and April, 1983. Philadelphia.
    4. ANSI/ASTM F803-83 Standard Specification for Eye Protectors for Use by Players of Racquet Sports. Philadelphia.

Anonymous
    1969   *Man, Sweat, and Performance*. Rutherford, New Jersey: Becton, Dickinson and Co.
    1977   Rowing Safety Rules for Coaches and Athletes. *The Oarsman* 9(1):20.

Appenzeller, H.
    1978   *Physical Education and the Law*. Charlottesville, VA; The Michie Company.

Armstrong, R., and W. Tucker
    1964   *Injury in Sports*. Springfield, Illinois: Charles C. Thomas.

Ashworth, K.
    1985   Athletic Injury Prevention: Safety Against Horror Stories Convention Report. *PEPI Newsletter*, February.

Baley, J.A., and D.L. Matthews
    1984   *Law and Liability in Athletics, Physical Education, and Recreation*. Newton, Massachusetts: Allyn and Bacon.

Barrell, G., P. Cooper, A. Elkington, J. MacFadyen, R. Powerll, and P. Tormey
    1981   Squash Ball to Eye Ball: the Likelihood of Squash Players Incurring an Eye Injury. *British Medical Journal* 92:893-895.

Batterman, C.
    1968   *The Techniques of Springboard Diving*. Cambridge: The MIT Press.

Bishop, J.B., R.W. Norman, R. Wells, D. Ranney, and B. Skleryk
    1983   Changes in the c of m and icm of a Headform Induced by a Hockey Helmet and Face Shield. *Canadian Journal of Sports Sciences* 8(1).

Brahatcek vs. Millard School District 202 Number 86, 273 NW, 2nd 680 (1979)

Burke, E.
    1986   *The Science of Cycling*. Champaign, IL: Human Kinetics.

Burch, G., and N. Depasquale
    1962   *Hot Climates, Man and His Heart*. Springfield, Illinois: Thomas Brooks.

Buskirk, E.R.
    1968   Problems Related to Conduct of Athletes in Hot Environments. *Physiological Aspects of Sports and Physical Fitness*. B. Balke, ed. Chicago, IL: The Athlete Institute.

Canadian Standards Association
    1982   The Quest for Safety in Canadian Sports, 1982. Toronto, Canada.
    n.d.1   Face Protectors for Ice Hockey and Lacrosse Players, C.S.A. Z262/2-M78. Toronto, Canada.
    n.d.2   National Standards of Canada. Hockey Helmets C.S.A. 262.1-1975 revised to CAN 3 Z262.1M83. Ontario, Canada.

Castaldi, C.R.
    1981   Injuries to the Teeth. Pages 147-157 in: *Sports Injuries: The Unthwarted Epidemic*. P.F. Vinger and E.F. Hoerner, eds. Littleton, Massachusetts: PSG Publishing Co.

Channing vs West Valley School District, Yakima County, WA. 1984.

Christensen, C., and K. Clarke
    1983   Fourth Annual Catastrophic Injury Report 1981-1982. Vienna, VA: U.S. Gymnastics Safety Association.

Clement, A.
    1987   Educational Malpractice: Physical Educators Should Be Concerned. In Press. *The Physical Educator*.

Clemett, R., and S. Fairhurst
    1980   Head Injuries in Squash: A Perspective Study. *New Zealand Medical Journal* 92:1-3.

Collins, M.
    1976   How to Combat Hypothermia. *The Oarsman* 8(4)34.

Connors, E.T.
    1981   *Educational Tort Liability and Malpractice*. Bloomington, ID: Phi Delta Kappa.

Consumer Product Safety Commission (CPSC)
    1977   *Medical Analysis of Swimming Pool Injuries*. Washington, D.C.: Consumer Product Safety Commission.
    1981   Overview of Sports Related Injuries to Persons 5-14 Years of Age. Washington, D.C.

Council on National Cooperation in Aquatics (CNCA)
    1975   *Swimming Pools: A Guide to their Planning, Design, and Operation*. Fort Lauderdale, FL: Hoffman Publications, Inc.

Damron, D.F.
    1981   Injury Surveillance Systems for Sports. Chapter I in: *Sports Injuries: The Unthwarted Epidemic*. P.F. Vinger and E.F. Hoerner, eds. Littleton, Massachusetts: PSG Publishing Co.

Davis, K., and R. McFeters
    1974   Care of Neck and Back Injuries Following Diving Accidents. *Journal of Health, Physical Education, and Recreation*. May, pp. 69-71.

DeMers, G.
    1983   Head-splint Rescue for Aquatic Related Neck Injuries. *Journal of Physical Education, Recreation, and Dance*. October, pp. 66-67.

Dibortolo vs. Metropolitan School District of Washington Township, 440 N.E. 2d 506 (1982).

Easterbrook, M.
    1982   Eye Injuries in Squash and Racquetball Players: An Update. *The Physician and Sportsmedicine* 10(3):47-56.

Elam, R.P.
    1981   *Oregon State University Football Summer Conditioning Program*. Corvallis, Oregon: Oregon State University.

Fox, E.L.
    1979   *Sports Physiology*. Philadelphia: W.B. Saunders Co.

George, G. (Ed.)
    1985   *USGF Gymnastics Safety Manual*, United States Gymnastics Federation, Indianapolis, IN.

Gabrielsen, M.
    1980   Spinal Cord Injuries Resulting from Diving. *Aquatics in the 80's*. A Report of the 21st National Conference. Manassas, VA: Council of National Cooperation in Aquatics.
    1981   *Diving Injuries: Prevention of the Most Catastrophic Sport Related Injuries*. Indiana, PA: Council on National Cooperation in Aquatics.

Haugen, R.K.
    1963   The Cafe Coronary: Sudden Death in Restaurants. *Journal of the American Medical Society* 186:142-143.

Hayes, D.
    1977   Effects of Intraoral Mouthguards on Ventilation. *Physician and Sportsmedicine*, January, pp. 61-66.

Henderson, D.H.
    1985   Physical Education Teachers. *Journal of Physical Education, Recreation, and Dance*, February, Vol. 56:44-48.

Henderson, J.
    1973   *Emergency Medical Guide*. Third Edition. New York: McGraw-Hill Book Co.

Hooks, G.
1974   *Weight Training in Athletics and Physical Education.* New Jersey: Prentice-Hall, Inc.
Ingram D., and J. Lewkonia
1973   Ocular Hazards of Playing Squash Rackets. *British Journal of Opthalmology* 57:434-437.
Insurance Company of North America
1984   *Loss Control for School Athletic Injuries.* Bulletin.
Keeton, W.P. (Ed.)
1984   *Prosser and Keeton on the Law of Tort.* St. Paul, MN: West Publishing Company.
Kemp, M.
n.d.   Here's the Basic Concept for Ice Hockey. Madison, Wisconsin: Athletic Purchasing and Facilities.
Klafs, C.E., and D. Arnheim
1981   *Modern Principles of Athletic Training.* Fifth Edition. St. Louis: C.V. Mosby Co.
Korpela, E.
1985   Tort Liability of Public Schools and Institutions of Higher Learning for Accidents Occurring in Physical Education Classes, *American Law Reports, 3rd.* Rochester, N.Y.: The Lawyers Co-Operative Publishing Company, 361-391.
LaBonne, M.
1980   "Eye Injuries: Always Serious." *Racquetball*, pp. 23-24. June.
1983   "Racquetsports eye injuries: They don't call it "squash" for nothing." *Executive Fitness Newsletters*, pp. 7, 14. April.
Larson v. Independent School District No. 314, Brahan, Minnesota, 289 N.W. 2d 112 (1979) (Rehearing denied, 1980).
Leibee, H.
1965   *Tort Liability for Injuries to Pupils.* Campus Publishers.
1971   School Law and Legal Liability. *Administration of Athletics in Colleges and Universities,* American Alliance of Health, Physical Education, Recreation and Dance.
Lueck v. City of Janesville, 57 Sisc. 2d 254, 204 N.W. 2d 6 (1973).
Maglischo, E.
1982   *Swimming Faster.* Palo Alto, CA: Mayfield Publishing Co.
Mathews, D.K., and E.J. Fox
1976   *The Physiological Basis of Physical Education and Athletics.* Second Edition. Philadelphia, London, and Toronto: W.B. Saunders Co.
McPatchie, G.
1982   *Injuries in Combat Sports.* Offox Press, Oxford.
Mirkin, G., and M. Hoffman
1978   *The Sports Medicine Book.* Boston: Little, Brown and Co.
Mueller, F.O., and C.S. Blyth
1984-5   Third Annual Report, National Center for Catastrophic Sports Injury Research, University of North Carolina, Chapel Hill, NC.
Murphy, R.J., and W.F. Ash
1965   Prevention of Heat Illness in Football Players. *Journal of the American Medical Association* 194:650-654.
National Association for Girls and Women in Sport, *1984 Gymnastics Guide,* Reston, VA; AAHPERD.
National Federation of State High School Associations, 1986-97 Officials NF
1986   Basketball Rule Book. Kansas City, MO.
Nelson, R., and H. Berger
1971   *Handball.* Englewood Cliffs, N.J.: Prentice-Hall Sport Series.
Northcote, R., A. Evans, and D. Ballantine
1984   Sudden Death in Squash Players. *The Lancet.* Jan. 21:148-150.
O'Shea, J.P.
1979   *Scientific Prinicples and Methods of Strength Fitness.* First Edition. Reading, Massachusetts: Addison-Wesley Publishing Co.
Pashby, T.J.
1981   Eye Injuries in Hockey. *International Opthalmology Clinics* 21:59.
Roberson, R., and H. Olson
1969   *Beginning Handball.* Belmont, CA: Wadsworth Sport Skills Series.
Schmidt, R.
1975   Karate. *Medicine and Science in Sports* 7(1):59-61.
Scrivener, A.
1973   Impact-Resistant Lenses. *British Journal of Physiological Optics* 28:26-33.
Shepard, G.
1977   *Bigger Faster Stronger.* Second Edition. Salt Lake City, UT: Hawks Publishing Co.
Smith v. Vernon Parish School Board, 442 S. 2d 1319 (La. App. 3d Civ. 1983).
Southmayd, W., and H. Hoffman
1981   *Sportshealth.* New York, NY: Quick Fox.

Strandemo, S.
    1980   "For a better game—game out of the way." *National Racquetball*, March.
    —   Total Racquetball, San Diego, CA: Ektelon, 70-77
Strauss, R.H., ed.
    1979   *Sports Medicine and Physiology*. Philadelphia, PA: W.B. Saunders Co.
Tunstall, P.
    1984   Sudden Death and Sport-Preventable or Inevitable? *British Journal of Sports Medicine* 18(4):293-294.
United States Military Academy
    1979   *Instructor Handbook-Handball*. West Point, NY: Publication of Department of Physical Education.
Vinger, P.F.
    1983   "Eye protection for racquet sports." *Journal of Physical Education, Recreation and Dance*. June. pp.46-48, 54. (extensive bibliography)
Washington State Public Health Association (WSPHA)
    n.d.   *Swimming Pool Operation: A Manual for Operators*. Seattle, WA: Washington State Public Health Association.
Wilmore, J.
    1982   *Training for Sport and Activity: The Physiological Basis of the Conditioning Process*. Boston, MA: Allyn and Bacon.
Wyness, G., and E. Long
    1985   Dealing with the Specter of Catastrophic Injuries. *Athletic Business*, January:36-39.
Yessis, M.
    1977   *Handball*. Third Edition. Dubuque, IA: W.W. Brown Co.
Yubic, T.
    1972   *Handball*. Philadelphia, PA: W.B. Saunders Co.